Dedication

This book is a milestone in a long journey that started with a silly Border Collie / Great Pyrenees mix who changed my world. I dedicate this book to my dog, Rodrigo, without whom none of this would be happening. Because of his health issues, I turned my blogging world upside down as I first tried to find a cure for my dog and then, once I found the answer, share the benefits of raw feeding to the world.

I dedicate this book to Blue aka Blueberry. The dog that I was compelled to adopt and fell in love with immediately. This Angel joined our family for a short time to teach me to appreciate the moment and stay focused on my goals.

To Sydney, who is my canine doppleganger, always by my side, trusting me to do what's best for her.

To Scout and Zoey, two sweet souls who, together, brought Blue's spirit back into our home to help mend our broken hearts.

And finally to Johan, the man who said, “ookaayyy,” when I announced that I was going to feed the dogs raw meat. Johan has patiently supported me through epic meltdowns when I broke my website, a wounded ego when a friend became a troll, and face splitting smiles at every win. Thank you for knowing that the path to my heart is a new tool to add to my raw feeding arsenal. Best Christmas and Birthday presents ever!

Forward

Six years ago, a veterinarian told my human that I would live a short life because I wasn't feeling so hot. My veterinarian recommended a food that raised red flags, inspiring my human to start a journey that led her to start a blog and write this book. Today, I no longer have the joint issues, allergies, and digestive issues that prompted many veterinarian appointments and lots of medication.

I'm a happy, healthy dog because my human followed her gut instead of following the advice of a veterinarian that she felt was wrong.

Kimberly wrote this book because she knows that I'm not the only dog living with health issues. She understands that dogs can survive on kibble, but they thrive on a diet of raw dog food. And she wanted to create a roadmap to help guide others to the path we have walked for four years.

After helping me and my sister, Sydney, my human now helps other dogs and their humans.

In this book, you'll learn about our journey into raw feeding and how my mommy was able to heal my gut and Sydney's joints through a biologically appropriate diet.

- You'll learn why she doesn't worry about bacteria in raw dog food.
  - You'll learn what supplements she adds to our food.
  - You'll learn why she allows us to choose the proteins we eat.
  - And a lot more.

You can read it from the beginning to the end or you can bounce around and read what captures your eye in the table of contents.

This book was written for people who are in a similar spot that my human found herself in four years ago. She had a young dog that wasn't thriving (that's me) and began the search for an answer. She was trying to learn how to help me in a community where the information was overwhelming and confusing. She loved me enough to keep learning and today, I'm living proof that raw feeding is the answer.

Rodrigo "Knock it Off" Gauthier

An Introduction to Raw Feeding

My name is Kimberly, I have four dogs, and I'm a raw feeder.

In 2013, I worked with Darwin's Pet to transition my dogs to a raw food diet. I was nervous about the cost and I didn't understand anything about dog nutrition. I knew that my dog, Rodrigo, was suffering from a myriad of health issues because of dry dog food and I prayed that raw dog food was the answer.

Today, more than four years later, Rodrigo is a healthy 7-year-old dog. We were joking recently about waltzing Rodrigo down to the vet clinic where his first vet predicted that our dog would live a short life due to his health issues. It would be worth the trip if we could change the vet's mind about raw feeding. He'd probably have us arrested for trespassing.

Rebooting Raw Feeding from A to Z

This year, I hosted my first workshops teaching others how to make dog food. I wasn't able to lease a kitchen space, so I cooked dog food and thawed raw dog food to bring to the workshops, along with supplements, treats, and copies of my Quick Start Guide to Raw Feeding.

I had a blast talking to people, answering questions, and sharing our story. The workshop was the boost I needed to begin writing the updated version of my book Raw Feeding from A to Z.

I wrote and published my first A to Z series in April 2014 on my blog, Keep the Tail Wagging®. In this book, A Novice's Guide to Raw Feeding, you will find a guide to transitioning to raw feeding, information about raw feeding using the alphabet as a guide, and raw dog food recipes that work for my dogs.

Three years ago, I thought raw feeding was too expensive; today, I buy 99% of my supplies through a local raw food co-op, which cut my monthly budget by more than 50%. Three years ago, I thought raw feeding was too complicated; today, I find raw feeding easier than feeding kibble. I wrote this book to make raw feeding easier for other dog owners. Enjoy.

Why I Feed My Dogs Raw Dog Food

When I switched to raw, it was to give Rodrigo relief from environmental allergies, food allergies, ear infections, chronic diarrhea, skin rashes, itchy paws, and joint pain. Today, I understand that we feed raw because it's species appropriate. A diet filled with highly processed foods were the cause of my dog's health issues.

The first two weeks of feeding raw we saw a huge improvement to Rodrigo's health, and he and my other dogs only ate raw in the morning; we fed them kibble in the evening during a transition period of three months. The addition of fresh foods to a diet of processed foods made a significant difference.

Note: We did not mix raw and kibble together; this would have been too much for Rodrigo's gut as the two diets battled it out (they have different pH levels). I later learned that transitioning our dogs over three months wasn't necessary. It was recommended because of my concern over the cost of premade raw, which can be overwhelming when raising multiple dogs.

Why I Write About Raw Feeding

The reason I write about raw feeding is to let others know the importance of adding fresh food to our dogs' diet. I want others to see the amazing transformations like what I witnessed with Rodrigo.

When I became a raw feeder and started researching dog nutrition, I found it complicated, contradictory, and overwhelming. One person told me that yogurt was great for dogs; another person told me yogurt is bad for dogs. Some raw feeding groups are welcoming of all models of raw feeding, while others ban the mention of vegetables.

I write about raw feeding because the raw feeding community is all that many pet lovers have and I feel that it's my responsibility to share my experiences, paying forward the time others have taken to share their experience and knowledge with me.

Quick Start Guide to Raw Feeding

Transitioning a Dog to a Raw Food Diet

There are many paths to take for people who want to transition their dog to raw dog food; below is what I recommend based on my experience with my dogs and what I've learned over the past four years from other raw feeders and leaders in the raw feeding community.

1 – Start Educating Yourself About Raw Feeding

The most important step is to start educating yourself about raw feeding. Join raw feeding groups, watch YouTube videos, connect with a pro-raw veterinarian and local raw feeders, and pick up a few books. Don't allow your education to come from one place because many of us are self-taught and what works for my dogs may not work for your dogs. Instead, soak up as much knowledge from as many sources as possible so that you're prepared to meet your dogs' needs.

2 – Start with a Quality Premade Raw Brand

I'm a fan girl of Darwin's Natural Pet Food; this is the brand that helped me transition my dogs to raw in 2013. A customer service representative from Darwin's Pet will walk you through setting up your first order and best practices for introducing raw to your dog. This is the easiest way to transition because the balancing, sourcing, and delivery are taken care of for you.

Of course, you'll pay for that amazing service too. If your budget is tight, joining a raw food co-op and sourcing from hunters, farmers, and people looking to clean out their freezers is an option.

The following are brands that I feed to my dogs.

- Darwin's Natural Pet Food (lamb, bison tripe)
- Answer's Pet Food (fermented fish stock, kefir, goat's milk)

- Raw Paws Pet Food (offers specials and free shipping)
- Columbia River Pet Food (quail, pheasant)
- Vital Essentials Raw (pork, cat food and treats)
- Primal Pet Food (sardine chubs)
- Northwest Naturals (lamb, vegetables)

You can buy premade raw online, at your local pet store, or through a raw food co-op.

Although premade raw is expensive, starting with premade raw allows a dog parent to quickly transition their dog to a balanced raw diet while giving them time to research recipes, sourcing, storage, and budget.

3 – Look for Sourcing in Your Area

If your budget is tight, then you'll have to become a DIY raw feeder, and that's where you want to be anyway. I still feed my dogs some premade raw brands. However, most of the food I buy is from a local meat supplier and I mix their meals twice a month while watching a movie or listening to a book.

To get started, you'll need to find sourcing in your area:

- Look for a meat supplier, butcher, farmer, or hunter in your area; make sure your local laws allow you to buy from hunters (this isn't legal in every state).
- Look to see if there is a raw food co-op in your area; this is a group of people who buy in bulk together at discounted prices.
- Check prices and connect with the meat manager at your local grocery store and Asian market.

Once you secure sourcing that meets your budget, you can move on to transitioning your dog to raw feeding.

4 – Introduce Raw Slowly to Your Dog

One mistake I made was to introduce my dogs to too many proteins and other ingredients too soon. It resulted in diarrhea for two days and me running back to kibble with my tail between my legs.

I also made a call to Darwin's Pet.

What I suggest is introducing a dog slowly. Don't worry about creating a balanced diet. Balance doesn't mean the same thing it did when we fed kibble. Raw feeders balance over time; for now, you want to focus on introducing your dog to raw.

WEEK ONE: Start with chicken or another white meat. Chicken is a great place to start because it's easy to digest, it's inexpensive and easy to source (locate). Alternatives to chicken include duck, turkey, guinea hen, pheasant, and quail.

- **Feeding Ground?** You can choose any cut of chicken that will go through your meat grinder. It's important to note that grinding bone voids some grinder warranties.
- **Feeding Whole?** Feed a raw meaty bone that is appropriate for your dog's size. If you have a small dog, start with a chicken wing or chicken thigh. If you have a large dog, start with a chicken quarter.

The purpose of feeding your dog this way is to allow their system to adjust to his/her new diet. Yes, feeding one cut of meat isn't a balanced diet, but we're not focusing on balance now, we're focusing on an introduction. Your initial week (or so) of feeding raw meaty bones is 100x better than feeding kibble.

If your dog is inhaling the raw meaty bones, try holding them while s/he eats; this will teach your dog to slow down. Or feed your dog ground raw in a slow feeding dog dish.

WEEK TWO: Introduce another protein; red meat is a good option. Once your dog seems to have a good handle on eating raw meaty bones, introduce another protein. Allow your dog to adjust to this meal change. Remember, don't feel the need to rush your dog. Allow him/her to gradually get used to the new diet; just because I say "week two" here doesn't mean that you have to switch if your dog isn't ready.

WEEK THREE: Introduce organ meat (offal and liver). If your dog doesn't like the texture of the organ meat, try mixing it into a vegetable blend or ground meat (not from a grocery store). Remember, the heart isn't an organ in raw feeding. You want to look for liver, pancreas, spleen, or kidneys (or all of these).

And one more time, don't worry about feeding a balanced diet at this time. Personally, I believe that the idea of a "balanced diet" was created by the kibble brands who needed to create balance to meet AAFCO standards; raw feeders don't have to meet those standards!

Feeding Guidelines…
When your dog is ready, you can attempt to transition to a more balanced diet with the understanding that you balance over time, not always in every meal or every day.

There are many raw food calculators online that take your dog's weight and activity level and tell you how much you should feed your dog per day. I weigh my dogs' meals to avoid overfeeding them (a past bad habit of mine). A general guideline is:

- Feed 2% of a dog's body weight to help them lose weight or for low activity dogs.
- Feed 2.5% of a dog's body weight to help them maintain weight.
- Feed 3% or more of a dog's body weight for active dogs.

5 – Monitor Your Dog's Stool

Four years later and I'm still monitoring my dogs' poop because it tells me how my dogs are doing and what I need to change about their diet. Monitoring your dog's stool during the transition to raw feeding will do the same. I love the idea of feeding my dogs a balanced raw diet, and I work hard to attain some balance. I follow the 80/10/5/5 while keeping in mind that my dogs have individual needs and what's "balanced" for one dog may not be for another. So I don't tear my hair out trying to make their diet perfect. Instead, I treat the 80/10/5/5 as a starting point.

Learning from My Dog's Stool

What I want to see is small, solid poops, however, this isn't always the case. The following are what I see with my dogs and how I correct their diet.

- White, Hard Poop: too much bone; increase muscle meat and/or organ meat.
- Soft Poop: too much organ meat; add more raw meaty bones.
- Soft Poop: reaction to a new protein; add Olewo carrots or, if it's a protein intolerance, stop feeding the meat.

These are just a few examples. As you become familiar with your dog's poop, you'll be able to identify what's happening and make quick adjustments.

LET YOUR DOG TELL YOU WHAT TO FEED

You may find that there are proteins that your dog loves and others that your dog turns away from; this is okay. Alternating proteins weekly or on another steady schedule will keep your dog engaged in their meal (eating the same thing daily gets boring) while allowing you to determine which foods do and do not work for your dog.

WHAT TO FEED A DOG

Muscle Meat	**Raw Bones**	**Liver**	**Offal**
80%	**10%**	**5%**	**5%**
e.g. Venison, Lamb, Goat, Rabbit, Pheasant, Quail, Duck, Elk, Emu	**e.g. Duck Necks, Lamb Necks**	**Liver**	**e.g. Pancreas, Spleen, Kidneys**

The above chart represents foods that I feed to my dogs; there are many more options available.

HOW MUCH RAW TO FEED A DOG

There are many raw food calculators online and this is a great place to start, however it's important to remember that each dog is different and while 2% may be a maintenance level for one dog, it could leave another dog constantly hungry.

Dogs are fed 2-4% of their body weight per day, split between two meals. Puppies are feed 10% of their current body weight or 3% of their estimated adult body weight per day, split between three meals.

Below is a graph using my dogs as an example:

Dog	Weight	Feed (pounds)	Feed (ounces)	Percentage	
Rodrigo	**~ 63 lbs.**	**2.05 lbs. per day**	**32.8 oz.**	**3.2%**	**Maintain Weight**
Sydney	**~ 75 lbs.**	**1.5 lbs. per day**	**24.0 oz.**	**2.0%**	**Lose Weight**
Scout	**~ 72 lbs.**	**2.16 lbs. per day**	**34.6 oz.**	**3.0%**	**Maintain Weight**
Zoey	**~ 63 lbs.**	**1.5 lbs. per day**	**24.0 oz.**	**2.3%**	**Lose Weight**

If you find that your dog is gaining too much weight or losing too much weight, adjust how much you are feeding.

HOW MANY TIMES OF DAY TO FEED A DOG

Puppies should be fed three times a day until they are 6 months old. Because we work full time, we hired a pet sitter to feed our dogs when they were puppies the puppies (10% of their body weight) until they were four months old when we switched to two meals per day

Adult dogs can be fed once or twice a day; some raw feeders also fast their dogs on a schedule.

Feeding Once a Day: Feeding a dog once a day eliminates the need to have a "fasting" day.

Feeding Twice a Day: This seems to be most common when feeding dogs; I feed my dogs in 12 hour intervals.

Benefits of Fasting: Some raw feeders fast their dogs weekly (or another set schedule) or naturally by feeding once a day. Fasting allows the gut to take a break from constantly digesting food. Allows the body to heal itself, which is why fasting is recommended when a dog has diarrhea. And fasting increases microphage levels to destroy harmful bacteria, viruses, and toxins.

Some Dogs Go Through a Detox

Some dogs experience a detox period once switched to raw food. Dog owners share that their dogs start shedding a lot, have mucus covered stool, and other mild symptoms that make them nervous about raw. Before freaking out and racing to the vet, ask yourself if your dog's behavior has changed (is s/he acting sick?) and double check the symptoms of detox others have reported. They tend to last a few days to a couple of weeks.

- mucus coating your dog's poop
- dry skin
- excess shedding
- runny eyes
- skin conditions may worsen before improving

While this may be unnerving, a detox period is the system's way of ridding excess toxins and other unhealthy things after being on a kibble diet. If you are worried about the detox period, work with a holistic veterinarian who is experienced in raw feeding and dog nutrition.

Adding Supplements to a Raw Diet for Dogs

When you initially transition a dog to a raw food diet, I don't think it's a great idea to add supplements. You may be tempted to add things that other raw feeders tell you about; I made this mistake, and it made raw feeding too complicated and some supplements offset (canceled out) others.

Raw fed dogs have different requirements than kibble fed dogs. For instance, Rodrigo used to be on a joint supplement; today, he has no need for a joint supplement because I've added duck feet and beef trachea to his diet, both high in glucosamine. Only giving my dogs what they need has helped me to save money. Instead, gradually add supplements as you see a need. Ideally, your dog should be able to get most of what they need nutritionally from their raw diet, however, if you're unable to source everything through whole foods, then you may need to add a supplement, for example, if you can't get sardines, then add fish oil to your dog's diet.

My last bit of advice on the supplements is to go with quality, proven brands. Not every human supplement is good for dogs.

Books on Raw Feeding

- Unlocking the Canine Ancestral Diet: Healthier Dog Food the ABC Way, Steve Brown
- Raw and Natural Nutrition for Dogs, Revised Edition: The Definitive Guide to Homemade Meals, Lew Olson
- Canine Nutrigenomics: The New Science of Feeding Your Dog for Optimum Health, W. Jean Dodds, DVM
- Dr. Becker's Real Food for Healthy Dogs and Cats, Beth Taylor and Karen Shaw Becker, DVM
- Feed Your Best Friend Better: Easy, Nutritious Meals and Treats for Dogs, Rick Woodford
- Work Wonders: Feed Your Dog Raw Meaty Bones, Tom Lonsdale

Blogs and Websites on Raw Feeding

- Keep the Tail Wagging; http://www.keepthetailwagging.com/
- Perfectly Rawsome; http://perfectlyrawsome.com/
- RawFed.com; http://rawfed.com/myths/
- PreyModelRaw.com; http://www.preymodelraw.com/
- BARFWorld.com; http://www.barfworld.com/

Videos on Raw Feeding

- Dr. Karen Becker
- Dr. Judy Morgan
- Rodney Habib
- Kimberly Gauthier
- Scott Marshall aka Dog Dad

Raw Feeding Groups

- Raw Feeders "Kicked Out" Club
- Raw Feeding 101 - Learn to Feed Raw
- Raw Feeding University
- RawFeeding Rebels
- K9 Kitchen
- Worldwide Canine Welfare Community

Raw Feeding 101

Definition of Raw Feeding

Raw feeding is a diet that consists of a ratio of raw muscle meat, organ meat, and bone. Raw feeders believe that feeding a diet of raw dog food is species appropriate, meaning that it's what dogs are meant to eat. We are all aware that dogs have evolved from the Grey Wolf and raw feeding is an attempt to mimic a wolf's diet while taking into account sourcing of ingredients and how dogs have adapted over the centuries.

One reason we prefer raw feeding to kibble is because raw feeding has a longer history. What many people don't know is that kibble hasn't been around for very long. It was invented during World War II as a solution when aluminum (which was originally used for canned dog food) was redirected to the war efforts and pet food manufacturers had to think of something new for their customers. And that's why we have kibble.

Over the years, pet food manufacturers have found that they can make more money by using inferior ingredients (corn and other grains, meat by-products, cheap synthetic vitamins), call their food balanced, and when dogs got sick, they'd sell dog parents "prescription" food that acted as a bandage instead of a cure for health issues.

While pet food manufacturers are keeping our dogs sick with their food; raw feeding is curing many illnesses. Dogs are living longer, healthier lives when raw feeding is combined with minimal to no vaccinations and limited exposure to flea and tick chemicals and other toxins.

Ratio of Ingredients in a Raw Diet for Dogs: Raw dog food consists of approximately 80% raw muscle meat, 10% raw bone, 5% liver, and 5% offal (secreting organs like pancreas, spleen, testicles, ovaries, and kidneys).

Raw Feeding Models (Diets)

While everyone ultimately ends up feeding what is best for their individual dog, we all start from one of two main models of raw feeding: BARF and

PREY Model.

BARF MODEL OF RAW FEEDING

The BARF model of raw feeding is the most common and what we see in most premade raw brands. BARF is an acronym for Biologically Appropriate Raw Food or Bones and Raw Food. The BARF model of raw feeding consists of raw muscle meat, raw bone, raw organ meat, raw fruits and vegetables, and other natural supplements.

Proponents of the BARF model of raw feeding feel that all ingredients in a natural, BARF diet offer our dogs vitamins, minerals, healthy fats, antioxidants and more.

Critics of the BARF model of raw feeding feel that adding produce is unnecessary and serves as a filler or, possibly, fiber. Some feel that dogs aren't capable of breaking down a diet heavy in fruits and vegetables due to the cellulose wall that acts as a barrier, preventing dogs from being able to absorb the nutrients. And some raw feeders believe that the process of breaking down the vegetables in a dog's system places stress on the pancreas and can lead to pancreatitis.

Although the BARF model can be fed whole, many times we see it fed as a ground diet to dogs.

Ratio of Ingredients in the BARF model of raw feeding: many times, you'll find that the BARF model calls for a reduction of the muscle meat to account for the fruits and vegetables: 65%-75% muscle meat instead of 80%, 10% raw bone, 5% liver, and 5% offal (secreting organs like pancreas, spleen, testicles, ovaries, and kidneys).

PREY MODEL OF RAW FEEDING

The PREY model of raw feeding leans towards feeding the whole animal and focuses on food sources for supplements, for example, if your dog needs a joint supplement, feed him cuts of meat high in chondroitin and glucosamine (e.g., duck feet).

While Prey model raw feeding seems to follow the diet of a wolf more closely than the BARF model, PMR (prey model raw) followers do add supplements when necessary and may use vegetables for weight loss and herbs for medicinal purposes when needed.

There is also a question of whether wolves eat the stomach contents of their vegetarian prey. Some believe that wolves shake out the stomach contents, only eating the meat, while others feel that wolves eat the whole animal, including the animal's last vegetarian meal. The theory that wolves shake out the stomach contents is based on a 40-year study by L. David Mech who lived with and observed wolves, documenting his findings in two books:

- Wolves on the Hunt
- Wolves Behavior and Ecology

Critiques of the Prey Model of raw feeding believe that the attempt to feed dogs like wolves is impossible. Wolves don't source their meat from the grocery store or butcher. Dogs today, while similar to their ancestor, now experience constant exposure to toxins (vaccinations, flea and tick treatments, cleaning products, etc.) — the antioxidants in vegetables, especially fermented vegetables, are beneficial to today's dogs.

Ratio of Ingredients in the Prey model of raw feeding: 80% muscle meat, 10% raw bone, 5% liver, and 5% offal (secreting organs like pancreas, spleen, testicles, ovaries, and kidneys).

Why Kibble isn't Good for Dogs (or Cats)

Kibble is an over-processed, repeatedly baked food that has lost all nutritional value so brands add in a bucket load of synthetic vitamins that are bought in a mix, preservatives to allow the food to sit in a warehouse for months on end, and a chemical based "natural flavor" to make the food appeal to dogs.

Kibble lacks moisture, leading to a constant state of dehydration and digestive issues. Because the digestive system is closely tied to the immune system, a diet of kibble will leave some dogs with poor health, like my Rodrigo, or worse.

THE MEAT AS THE FIRST INGREDIENT MYTH

We've been told to look for meat as the first ingredient, but this isn't a sign of a "quality" kibble. For instance, one of the leading kibble brands offers the following on their first line of ingredients: *Deboned Chicken, Chicken Meal (source of Glucosamine), Turkey Meal, Peas, Pea Protein, and Chicken Fat (preserved with Mixed Tocopherols).*

- The deboned chicken has water and, of course, water adds weight. The reason "deboned chicken" is first is because of the water, not the chicken.

- Chicken meal is chicken with the water removed, but in this food, they are using the meal as a source of glucosamine because the meal is mostly chicken bone and cartilage, not chicken meat.

- Turkey meal is the THIRD ingredient, which means that there is more water (deboned chicken) and bone (chicken meal) than turkey in this food.

- The brand adds peas and pea protein to boost the protein amount.

- Chicken fat causes the kibble to go bad faster; once the bag is opened, the fat begins to oxidize. And guess what! Transferring the food to a plastic container will make it go bad even faster; the dog food bags are made from products that slow oxidation, plastic containers are not.

It's all a crock.

We know that people need real, whole, minimally processed foods in order to thrive. As humans, if making healthy eating choices has improved our health, it shouldn't take a leap to realize that this same logic applies to our dogs and cats.

Our dogs are meant to eat a diet of raw muscle meat, bone, and organs, despite what the traditional veterinarian community and the big pet food companies are trying to tell us. What did dogs eat before commercial can and dry dog food hit store shelves? They ate what we ate along with a diet of raw meat; i.e., a diet high in vitamins, minerals, antioxidants, healthy fats, living enzymes, and moisture.

As people, we are told that fewer processed foods, whole foods, and foods free of chemicals and additives are better for us; is it so hard to believe the same is true for our dogs?

LET YOUR DOG TELL YOU WHAT TO FEED

You may find that there are proteins that your dog loves and others that your dog turns away from; this is okay. Alternating proteins weekly or on another steady schedule will keep your dog engaged in their meal (eating the same thing daily gets boring) while allowing you to determine which foods do and do not work for your dog.

Common Fears About Raw Feeding

The veterinarian community has been consistently publishing misinformation about raw feeding in order to discourage people from feeding their pets a raw diet and I completely understand. I have had an opportunity to speak with a lot of veterinarians about raw feeding and many have cared for pets brought to them after being fed an improperly balanced raw diet.

However, raw feeding isn't the dangerous diet many would have us believe.

IS RAW FEEDING SAFE?

Absolutely! Yes, handling raw meat does expose us and our dogs to bacteria, however, proper food handling and hygiene practices is all we need to stay safe. If an inspiring raw feeder or a dog has a compromised immune system, raw feeding is still an option. Many premade raw brands make packaging that reduces exposure to raw meat when feeding our dogs.

High Pressure Pasteurization (HPP): HPP is a process that reduces pathogens in raw meat. HPP is a form of processing and some believe it destroys many nutrients in raw, however, it does make raw more accessible to dog owners who are concerned about the bacteria in a raw diet.

WILL THE BACTERIA IN RAW MAKE MY DOG SICK?

Nope! Unless your dog has a compromised immune system, raw is perfectly safe. A dog's system has several defenses against the bacteria in raw. Their saliva has properties that kill bacteria, their gut isn't very hospitable to bacteria, and their digestive tract is short and processes food quickly and efficiently.

If you are raising a dog with a compromised immune system, speak with a holistic vet who is experienced in raw feeding before crossing the diet off your list. If raw isn't an option, a home cooked diet may be best for your dog.

IS RAW DOG FOOD BALANCED?

Yes! A balanced raw diet consists of 80% muscle meat, 10% bone, 5% liver, and 5% offal. Premade raw brands, for the most part, offer a balanced raw diet. DIY (do-it-yourself) raw feeders can attain balance per meal, however, many find it easier to attain balance over time.

Because the raw feeding "trend" is on fire at the moment, we are seeing new brands come to market that are not providing a balanced diet. Some are combining too many proteins, skipping the offal (secreting organs like pancreas, kidneys, and spleen), and opting for a synthetic vitamin blend.

IS RAW FEEDING EXPENSIVE?

I would love to say, "No," raw feeding is cheaper than feeding kibble, however, it really depends on where you live, the resources available to you, and how much time you can commit to the diet. For instance, I spend 50% less money by making a balanced raw meal for my dogs than I did when I bought premade raw.

I feed a combination of DIY raw and premade raw, buying 99% of the food through a local raw food co-op and placing an order with Darwin's Pet every other month (lamb or bison green tripe). A raw food co-op is an organization that orders raw from meat suppliers, local farms, and pet food distributors at discounted prices. There is an annual membership fee, order frequency, and pick up dates. Co-ops are not the same as a raw food brand that delivers to your door.

Visit my blog to search for a raw food co-op in your area:
http://www.keepthetailwagging.com/coop

DO RAW FEEDERS MISTRUST VETERINARIANS?

Yes, and no. The first veterinarian who saw my puppies, Rodrigo and Sydney, was intolerant of questions, didn't like rescue dogs, and would not have been supportive of a raw food diet. In my experience, while many veterinarians don't support raw, they may get on board if you're able to demonstrate that you will do the research needed to learn how to feed your dog a balanced, raw diet.

Some raw feeders mistrust veterinarians because of the amount of misinformation being promoted via flyers and on social media about the dangers of raw. However, I do respect a veterinarians education. I prefer to work with veterinarians who have experienced with raw feeding or who will keep an open mind and support me when I share my choice to feed raw.

Finding the Right Raw Food Sources

WHAT TO LOOK FOR IN A RAW FOOD SOURCE

With the growing popularity of raw feeding, we're seeing a lot of new sources and premade raw brands. There are new brands that are selling meals that aren't balanced, over priced (4x higher) raw meals, and suspiciously sourced raw meals.

When I'm looking into a new source, I'm interested in the following:

- Where does the meat come from?
- Is it 3D or 4D (diseased, dying, down, or dead) meat?
- What was the animal fed? Grass? Grain?
- Was the animal subjected to hormones, antibiotics, or other chemicals?
- What is the cost? Per pound?

If it's a premade raw brand, I'm also interested in knowing the following:

- What are the ingredients?
- Are there proprietary (secret) ingredients or blends?
- Does the brand follow the 80/10/5/5 rule for balancing?

Balance, Bacteria, Behavior, and Raw Dog Food

Balancing a Raw Food Diet

One of the critiques raw feeders receive is that our diet isn't balanced. What people don't realize is that those of us who are making raw dog food at home don't balance our dogs' meals per meal or per day, we balance their diet over time.

I strive to feed my dogs 80% muscle meat, 10% bone, 5% liver, and 5% offal (secreting organs like pancreas, spleen, and kidneys). I mix in an organic vegetable mix that includes spinach, kale, collard greens, carrots with greens, parsley, celery, garlic (no, it's not toxic to dogs in small amounts), zucchini, apples, and blueberries, and bone broth. I add supplements as needed.

To calculate the ratio of ingredients, I start with a site called PerfectlyRawesome.com, which has a bone ratio chart. I usually start with 40 pounds of duck wings…

- Duck wings are 39% bone (15.6 pounds) and 60% meat (24.4 pounds).

- 15.6 pounds / 10% = 156 pounds of total meat/bone/offal/liver to make a "balanced" meal.

- 156 pounds x 80% = 124.8 of muscle meat; which means I need 100.4 additional meat, which I can get from venison trim, duck gizzards, and duck hearts.

- 156 x 10% = 15.6 / 2 = 7.8 pounds each of liver and offal blend (I usually use liver and a green tripe organ blend from GreenTripe.com).

While attempting to balance a dog's raw diet per meal is possible, I have chosen to balance my dogs' raw diet over time. I believe that the concept of providing a balanced meal is a hold over from kibble brands that need to provide balance to meet AAFCO standards (a voluntary organization responsible for enforcing laws and regulations surrounding the safety of animal feed). Since I don't eat a balanced diet daily, I no longer focus on feeding my dogs a balanced diet daily — and it makes life a lot easier.

Determining if Your Raw Fed Dog isHealthy

To make sure your dog is getting what s/he needs, you can do the following:

- **monitor their poop** — raw fed dogs have small, solid poop. The color may change based on what you're feeding (venison creates darker poop than duck), but the color shouldn't range too much.

- **pay attention to their appearance** — raw fed dogs have gorgeous, shiny coats, clean teeth, fresh breath, and clean ears.

- **annual blood panels** – I take my dogs to the vet annually for a blood draw and an a-okay from the vet that they're doing good or recommendations of what I need to adjust in their diet.

There are times when I can't gather all of the ingredients I need. When this happens, I do the best I can because I balance over time. If you aren't comfortable with this, you can add a nutrient blend or meal balancer to your dog's raw meals.

Bacteria in Raw Dog Food

Another warning we hear about raw feeding is the bacteria, which is thought to be a hazard to our dogs and their humans. What people who issue these warnings fail to understand is:

- raw feeders wash their hands regularly, we clean our kitchens from top to bottom, and we wash our dogs' dishes.

- the raw food that I order arrives frozen and lives in the freezer until I'm ready to prepare two weeks of raw meals (with partially thawed ingredients), which is then stored back in the freezer.

Dogs are designed to consume raw meat because it's species appropriate:

- the saliva of dogs kills bacteria with each bite because it contains an enzyme called lysozyme that kills harmful bacteria.

- a dog's digestive system is shorter and pushes through the food fast enough to prevent any surviving bacteria from setting up camp; but not so fast that our dogs' systems won't absorb the nutrients they need to be happy and healthy.

And for those who warn us that dogs will shed salmonella, remind them of all of the dry dog food recalls due to salmonella.

Behavior of Raw Fed Dogs

One of the benefits of raw feeding that I read about was an improvement in behavior. I've been told that the dogs that are anxious, reactive, and aggressive are dogs that are living in a constant state of inflammation due to being fed a kibble diet.

Sydney has always been a sweet dog, and this hasn't changed. Scout and Zoey started on a raw diet at six weeks of age; they were always happy. Rodrigo, on the other hand, has a reputation (with me) of being a dick sometimes and this has improved partially due to a raw food diet.

Rodrigo's pancreas isn't producing an appropriate amount of digestive enzymes. The subsequent GI (gastrointestinal) issues lead to a compromised immune system (food allergies, environmental allergies, ear infections), digestive issues (diarrhea, chronic loose stool, gas, stomach gurgling, constant hunger), and behavioral issues (anxiety, fear, reactivity, aggression).

Combining raw dog food with a pancreas supplement* cleared everything up and he's my sweet dog again. He can still be a dick (stealing toys, stealing treats, dominance humping), but he's easier to train, he has a better recall, and recently, he exhibited amazing self control. There were three horses and a dog on the trail that borders our property. He noticed them and came to me when I called and we went inside. The old Rodrigo would have run out to the trail to introduce himself.

* *All of my dogs now enjoy fermented foods instead of digestive supplements.*

Rodrigo, raw fed since 2013, is still a reactive dog, which we're addressing successfully with training. Zoey, raw fed nearly her entire life, is also reactive and anxious, which is being addressed with training and supplements (Ewegurt). All in all, our dogs are wonderful, well behaved (most of the time), and a joy to be around.

Cost, Calcium, Carnivores, and Raw Dog Food

Cost of Raw Feeding

When I wrote about the cost of raw feeding during the 2014 edition of Raw Feeding from A to Z, I was coming from the perspective of someone who didn't have a handle on ordering through a co-op. It took me a while to develop a solid routine. I've had two years to get used to ordering through the co-op, and on average, I spend about $250/month on dog food, treats, supplements, toys, and other supplies for four dogs (60 pounds to 75 pounds).

Over the years, I've found several other ways to save money on raw feeding:

- Make raw dog food at home; limit the purchase of premade raw dog food.
- Keep an eye out for other local raw feeders who want to sell or trade food in their freezer.
- Watch for specials offered by the co-op, Raw Paws Pet Food, and other pet brands.
- Become an Amazon Prime member to get free shipping on supplements and treats.
- Make homemade dog treats.

More ways to save money on raw feeding include:

- Buy trim from local butchers and hunters.
- Raise cattle, rabbits, and other animals for meat.
- Search Craigslist for people emptying freezers, or post a

Craigslist ad.

I do have pet insurance for my dogs, and because I invested when they were young and they're healthy, the premiums are still low. And, finally, my dogs go to the vet annually for a wellness check and occasionally (maybe one dog a year) for other care. Sydney enjoys acupuncture and chiropractic adjustments every other month.

Raw feeding costs less than feeding dry dog food because I no longer have regular vet appointments to treat health issues brought about by constant inflammation some dogs (aka Rodrigo) experience when whey are fed a kibble diet.

Speaking with raw feeders around the country, I now appreciate how lucky I am to have the resources available in Washington.

Calcium in Raw Dog Food

I feed our dogs a modified raw food diet based on the BARF Model that I call FrankenBARF. It is 80% muscle meat, 10% bone, and 5% liver, and 5% offal (secreting organs).

Along with the 80/10/5/5 ingredients, I add vegetables and supplements based on my dogs' needs.

One of the worries I had about making raw dog food was making sure my dogs received enough calcium. Several of the orders I place with the co-op are meat only: venison, elk, emu, and alpaca. I have two ways of adding calcium/bone to those meals:

- I use duck wings or duck necks as a base, mixing in an organ blend (DIY or from a brand) to create a balanced diet.
- I either add green tripe to their meal — it has a 1:1 calcium, phosphorous ratio — or feed the dogs green tripe for several meals during the week. For instance, they'll eat venison/organ blend five days during the week, and green tripe two days during the week.

I do not use bone meal in my dogs' food because most of the bone meal on the market is heat processed, making it difficult for dogs to digest. When I was looking for quality bone meals, I wasn't able to find any that were sourced in the US and provided details about the sourcing.

Are Dogs Carnivores or Omnivores?

Some people believe dogs are omnivores while others believe dogs are carnivores. I fall into the carnivore category because of their teeth (made for ripping meat from bone and chomping bone) and what I believe to be a species-appropriate diet — raw meat, raw bone, and raw offal/organ meat.

My opinion isn't based on science or studying wolves and dogs; it's based on my experience as a raw feeder. Therefore, I may be wrong, and I'm okay with being wrong. But I don't think I am. But I could be.

There is also a disagreement in the raw feeding community about whether dogs need fruits and vegetables. Here are my thoughts.

- I believe vegetables offer nutrients and antioxidants.
- I think vegetables can be medicinal, promote weight loss, or provide a nice snack.
- I believe dogs (at least my dogs) can consume vegetables without taxing their pancreas because I puree vegetables to break the cellular wall before feeding it to my dogs, or feed fermented vegetables. Feeding a BARF diet will not cause my dogs to have pancreatitis.

Feeding my dogs organic vegetables and fruit doesn't make them omnivores, it just makes them well-fed carnivores.

Disease, Dehydrated Food, and Dog Treats for Raw Fed Dogs

Diseases Cured by Raw Feeding

I'm not a veterinarian, so I'm not going to front and act like I know how to treat diseases in dogs. What I do know is that there are health issues that are improved or cured when dogs are fed a species-appropriate diet.

Working to understand Rodrigo's gut issues has taught me that the gut is closely connected to the immune system. When Rodrigo's gut wasn't healthy, he had:

- Daily loose stool, diarrhea, and gas
- Chronic ear infections
- Angry, red rashes on this back and tummy
- Itchy paws that he licked until sores developed
- Environmental and food allergies

Over the past few years, a combination of a species-appropriate diet, a quality digestive supplement, and feeding the right proteins has helped strengthen Rodrigo's gut, which has, in turn, strengthened his immune system.

Rodrigo hasn't had ear infections or rashes since I switched him to raw 4 years ago. He's stopped obsessively licking his paws shortly after being switched to raw dog food. And his poop is solid and small thanks to fermented foods (vegetables, fish stock, kefir) that help his body with digestive enzymes.

A few diseases that can be cured/improved with a raw diet include:

Diabetes – a raw food diet doesn't cause blood sugar spikes like kibble, which is higher in carb content. If you choose to feed BARF, you can select the lower glycemic vegetables and fruit if you're watching for blood sugar spikes. While raw may not cure your dog's diabetes, it will greatly improve your dog's health.

Pancreatitis or EPI – a raw food diet contains healthier fats and natural, living enzymes that can help a dog with pancreatitis or EPI. Rodrigo doesn't have EPI, however, I did try a pancreas supplement that helped his digestive issues immensely. After six months, I switched him to fermented foods which continued to keep his gut and immune system healthy.

Kidney Disease – dry dog food is the worst thing you can feed a dog with kidney disease; it's often made with inferior proteins, it's taxing on the kidneys because of all the synthetic ingredients, and it's dehydrating. On the other hand, a diet of fresh food is ideal for a dog with kidney failure because you can control the quality of protein you feed, a raw food diet is moisture rich, and there are no harsh/mystery ingredients.

Reducing protein isn't necessary for all animals with kidney disease; I recommend finding a holistic vet that is experienced in raw feeding who can help you build the right, species-appropriate diet.

Joint Health – a raw food diet isn't inflammatory like dry dog food; therefore, feeding raw improved my dogs joint health and reduced pain. Thanks to raw, Rodrigo went from a dog that wasn't putting weight on a leg to a dog that races around our property. Golden paste and Canine System Saver have been a successful addition to their diet.

Obesity – Rodrigo and Sydney were overweight when I switched them to a raw food diet. Rodrigo dropped 10 pounds in the first year. Sydney is currently on a diet; so far, she's lost 10 pounds and has 5 pounds to go. Feeding our dogs lean meats, healthy animal fats, and organic greens will lead to a healthier metabolism and immune system — which lead to a healthier weight.

Dental Health – I've been told by pet store employees and several veterinarians that kibble helps to clean a pet's teeth. Nothing could be further from the truth. Our dogs don't chew long enough for any teeth cleaning to happen and I have a $600 teeth cleaning bill to show you that they don't clean a cat's teeth either. What does clean my dogs' teeth is chewing on raw meaty bones and recreational bones; I brush my cat's teeth.

If your dog has an illness or disease, please speak with a holistic veterinarian experienced in raw and home-cooked diets for dogs to learn what you should feed your dog to help improve his/her health.

Dehydrated vs. Freeze-Dried Dog Food

A few years ago, I didn't understand the difference between dehydrated dog food and freeze-dried dog food. Today, when I hear the phrase "dehydrated raw," I giggle because if it's dehydrated, it's not raw.

When food is dehydrated, heat is used to evaporate the water from the ingredients. Although it's low heat, allowing many of the nutrients to remain intact, the food is still being cooked, and the cellular structure of the food is being altered.

With freeze-dried dog food, frozen food is put in a vacuum chamber in which the ice is evaporated. The temperature remains below freezing, and the nutrients remain intact. This is why I think freeze-dried dog food is superior to dehydrated. But both are miles better than commercial dry dog food.

Dehydrated and freeze-dried dog food is great as food toppers, convenient to feed when traveling, and an alternative for people who aren't ready (or able) to feed their dogs' a raw food diet.

Dog Treats for Raw Fed Dogs

Once I began paying attention to ingredients in my dogs' food, it didn't take long for me to become obsessed with their treats. The healthiest dog treats are the ones made at home with dog safe ingredients. I find dehydrating dog treats to be the easiest – I use one ingredient (sometimes two), I know the sourcing, and the dogs love their treats (I do too).

However, with my business schedule, it's easier to buy dog treats and the following is the criteria I follow to choose the healthiest dog treats for my pack.

- I look for limited ingredient dog treats due to Rodrigo's digestive issues; Scout and Zoe's and Vital Essentials Raw are my favorite brands for this reason.

- I avoid treats with potatoes.

- I look for treats with all natural ingredients.
- While I prefer protein treats for my dogs; Einstein Pets are our favorite "cookie" treats.

I purchase 95% of the treats my dogs eat through our local co-op. I subscribed to a monthly "chew" subscription box from RealPetFood.com.

There are a lot of dog treats that look healthy, but when you look at the ingredients, they're not so hot. The following ingredients are for dog treats that claim to be Trout and Pomegranate. Note where the main two ingredients fall (in weight) in the below list:

Peas, Sweet Potatoes, Vegetable Glycerin, Menhaden Fish Meal, Cane Molasses, Gelatin, **Trout, Pomegranate,** *Chicken Fat (Preserved with Citric Acid and Mixed Tocopherols), Natural Flavor, Rosemary Extract, Green Tea Extract.*

The only ingredients that I like are the sweet potatoes, trout, and pomegranate and if these were the only ingredients, mixed with chia or steel cut oats (maybe to hold them together), then I'd buy these treats. But my dogs don't need the peas, vegetable glycerin, fish meal, molasses, chicken fat, and natural flavor (which is not natural).

Although these treats won't harm my dogs, with so many healthy, natural dog treats on the market, there's no need for me to buy these treats.

Eggs, Education, Evidence, and Raw Feeding

Feeding Raw Eggs to Dogs

When I first started feeding a raw diet, people were shocked that I was adding raw eggs to my dogs' meals. Eggs will cause a biotin deficiency, eggs have salmonella, eggs will increase my dog's cholesterol levels.

Nope. Nope. NOPE!!!!

Eggs are GREAT for dogs. I feed them raw because cooking destroys all of the nutrients in eggs. Think about it, an egg is an incubator for a new life so the egg has a ton of vitamins and nutrients to grow the new life. I want my dogs to gain all that yumminess in their diet.

I prefer natural sources of vitamins for my dogs. Raw eggs add vitamins A, B2, B9, and B12, iron, selenium, and fatty acids to my dogs' raw diet.

- Vitamin A – eye sight, bone growth, and immune system
- Vitamin B2 – helps to convert food into fuel
- Vitamin B9 – formation of red blood cells, protein metabolism
- Vitamin B12 – nerve functions
- Iron – blood production and energy
- Selenium – behaves as an antioxidant in the body
- Fatty Acids – brain functions, skin and coat health, joints, and immune system

Egg Whites Only: I don't feed my dogs egg whites only; I think that's the source of the belief that dogs will develop a biotin deficiency. Some well-meaning dog lover probably fed their dogs egg whites only, because it's healthy for humans. I could totally see myself doing this too, but now I know better. Different species.

Feeding Raw Eggs to Dogs: I crack open the egg and add it to my dog's dish. I do count the weight of the egg when I'm measuring meals. I don't add the shell; three of my dogs won't eat it. I crack the yolk and mix it into the food for Sydney; the other three dogs like to lick the egg so I leave it on top.

Feeding Raw Egg Shells: Instead of adding the shell to my dogs' meals, I dry them out (or bake them for 10 minutes on low heat), grind them in my Nutri-Bullet, and sprinkle the egg dust over raw meals that don't contain bone. This is a great option for dogs that can't eat raw bone.

I only save the shells from eggs I get from friends (who have chickens) or local farms. Grocery store eggs have been rinsed with a chemical compound to make the eggs clean and pretty, so I don't feed my dogs those shells — better safe than sorry.

Before replacing raw bones with eggshells, it's important to understand that eggshells do not share the same calcium:phosphorus balance as raw bones. If you choose to use eggshells as an alternative to bones, consult with a veterinarian or nutritionist experienced in raw feeding.

Educating Ourselves About Raw Feeding

Many of us are learning how to feed our dogs a raw diet via the Internet and it's not easy. There is a lot of conflicting information out there and if you ask the wrong question, people grab the torches and troll you for days. There has got to be a better way, right?

- Join a raw feeding group — you will have to join a few to test them out and find the one that is right for you.

- Follow leaders in the Community – Dr. Karen Becker, Rodney Habib, Marty Becker, Susan Thixton, and many more people are sharing content daily about dog health and nutrition.

- Connect with local raw feeders — you can find them in groups, forums, and local raw food co-ops. Things began to click with me when I was able to sit down with someone to discuss raw feeding over coffee.

And, of course, there are a lot of books to read and a few blogs to follow. When you're searching Amazon, read the synopsis and the reviews to get an idea if it's the right book for you. The reviews on Amazon have saved me a lot of time and money.

MY FAVORITE BOOKS ARE:

- Raw Dog Food: Make It Easy for You and Your Dog Kindle Edition, by Carina Beth Macdonald

- The Barf Diet Kindle Edition, by Ian Billinghurst

- Raw and Natural Nutrition for Dogs: The Definitive Guide to Homemade Meals, by Lew Olson

- Dr. Becker's Real Food for Healthy Dogs and Cats, by Beth Taylor and Karen Shaw Becker DVM

MY FAVORITE MAGAZINES ARE:

- Dogs Naturally Magazine

- Healthful Dog UK (save 10% when you use the code KEEPTHETAILWAGGING10)

Dogs Naturally Magazine has an educational program. I completed the Pet Food Nutrition Specialist certification in December 2016. They also offer a Raw Pet Food certification.

Evidence that Raw Feeding is Beneficial for Dogs

One of the critiques we always get is that there is only anecdotal evidence that raw feeding is good for dogs. If we dismissed anecdotal evidence, we wouldn't have many of the advances we enjoy today. But for folks who need “proof” beyond the word of raw feeders around the globe, there are studies that show that fresh food is superior to processed foods.

- 2003 study conducted by Lippert and Sapy studied 500 dogs over a 5 year period — (http://www.ukrmb.co.uk/images/LippertSapySummary.pdf)

- 2005 study conducted at Purdue University on Scottish Terriers - (https://academic.oup.com/ilarjournal/article/55/1/100/847848/Urinar Bladder-Cancer-in-Dogs-a-Naturally/)

- 2016 New Zealand dog diet study a wake-up call for dog nutrition — (http://www.scoop.co.nz/stories/BU1703/S00534/new-zealand-dog-diet-study-a-wake-up-call-for-dog-nutrition.htm)

- On Going: Long Living Pets Projects - (https://longlivingpets.com/)

Plus, there are many veterinarians — also scientists — who support raw feeding. To find one, visit the AHVMA (American Holistic Veterinary Medical Association).

Fear, Fish Oil, Freezers, and Raw Feeding

Fear of Feeding Raw to Dogs

Many people who are new to raw feeding are scared out of their mind and I was one of them. It doesn't matter how many people told me that my dogs would be fine and raw feeding was easy, I didn't believe them. Not one of them.

I was afraid to feed my dogs raw because…

- I thought raw feeding would be complicated.
- I thought raw feeding would be expensive.
- I thought my vet would shame me for trying to kill my dogs.
- I thought my dogs would choke on a bone or break a tooth.

I stumbled for the first year as I learned about raw feeding. Connecting with other raw feeders and learning that I wasn't alone helped me get past my fears. Thanks to social media, I have a lot of great friends who feed raw. In fact, I met two of my best friends, Katrina and Tina, through social media and my blog. It's cool to be able to compare notes and ask random questions without the fear of being judged or made to feel stupid.

If you're afraid to take the plunge and transition your dog to a raw food diet, I suggest connecting with local raw feeders. Sometimes, talking with someone, one on one, and seeing how they feed their dogs helps you see that raw feeding isn't so scary.

Fish Oil for Raw Fed Dogs

Fish oil is great for skin/coat health, joint health (reverses inflammation), brain and neurological health, and heart health.

Dogs can't produce their own Omega 3 fatty acids, so they need to get it from their diet. There are three common types:

- ALA (α-linolenic acid): these are found in plants like hemp, camelina, and flaxseed.

- EPA (eicosapentaenoic acid) and DHA (docosahexaenoic acid): EPA and DHA partner together and come from sources like fish, eggs, and krill (the teeny fish that follow whales around)

I originally didn't think there was much of a difference between the ALA sources and the EPA/DHA sources, so I added Camelina Oil to the rotation when feeding my dogs. It's all Omega-3s, right? Yes, but they're not created equal. ALA needs to be converted to EPA/DHA in a dog's system. That's a lot of extra work when you can just give your dog fish oil that doesn't require the extra "conversion" step.

Other Sources of Omega 3s – I add raw eggs to my dogs' diet three days a week. I add sardines (canned in water or olive oil) to my dogs' raw meals two days a week. When I make salmon, I set aside some to share with the dogs (no bones); they love it.

I only add raw fish to my dogs' raw diet when I can split a fifty pound case with another raw feeder. Storage is limited despite having two freezers.

Freezers for Raw Fed Dogs

We have four dogs and one freezer that sits below the fridge in our kitchen and has zero extra space. When I started ordering in bulk, I purchased a 21 cubic foot freezer for $325 from the Appliance Recycling Outlet in Snohomish, Washington. Having dedicated freezer space for raw dog food allows me to buy in bulk, which has shaved 50% off of my monthly budget.

Today, I have two 21 cubic foot freezers.

I prefer to buy refurbished instead of used because a refurbished freezer has been serviced, may come with a warranty, and I'm confident that it works. I look for freezers with adjustable shelves, space in the door, and drawers at the bottom. Plenty of space for 200 pounds of raw dog food.

Gut Health, Green Tripe, Guidelines and Raw Feeding

Gut Health and Raw Feeding

Healthy Gut, Healthy Dog. This is the phrase that I think of when I think of Rodrigo. I started feeding a raw diet because Rodrigo had environmental allergies and food intolerances, chronic ear infections, skin rashes, itchy paws, and diarrhea and loose stool.

Food Allergies versus Food Intolerances: *a food allergy can be serious as it sparks an immune system reaction resulting in a multitude of symptoms. A food intolerance usually only impacts the gut.*

I wish that I understood that gut health was tied to immune system health, I would have realized that Rodrigo didn't need antibiotics every other month, he needed a probiotic. Maybe his gut health wouldn't have gotten so bad if I had known to soak his kibble in bone broth (loads of nutrients), add fresh vegetables (loads of nutrients), and add a digestive supplement.

Switching to raw helped Rodrigo. His rashes and ear infections went away immediately, but he still had itchy paws and three years of kibble had taken his toll on his gut so he continued to have GI issues. As a result of the lack of digestive enzymes, Rodrigo experienced the following:

- Continued weight loss despite always being hungry
- Pooping more often than the other dogs; his poop was larger, yellow or gray in color, and soft
- Eating his own poop (coprophagia)
- Increased gas and tummy noises
- Occasional diarrhea and vomiting

- Increased anxiety, fearful behavior

Rodrigo is now a healthy, raw fed dog.

Today, Rodrigo also eats fermented foods (vegetables, fish stock, kefir) to help his digestive system. He still has bigger poops than the other dogs, but they're a lot smaller than they were before (most days).

We don't stop at raw feeding; we make adjustments here and there to provide our dogs with what they need. Paying attention to my dog's behavior helped me narrow down what he was lacking in his diet and I was able to make an adjustment to improve his health.

Remember this mantra: **"Healthy Gut, Healthy Dog"**

Green Tripe and Raw Feeding

When I began feeding raw, I heard about the benefits of green tripe and set out to buy this magical food for my dogs. I ended up settling on canned green tripe because I couldn't find fresh green tripe.

What is Green Tripe?: green tripe is the stomach of ruminating animals like cows and bison.

Benefits of Green Tripe: I give our dogs green tripe because of the natural digestive enzymes, the perfect 1:1 calcium to phosphorous ratio and they love the taste and smell.

Not All Dogs Can Eat Green Tripe: I've found that green tripe doesn't work for Rodrigo unless I order through our raw food co-op or Darwin's Pet. I'm not 100% sure why that's the case. Green tripe gives Scout diarrhea when he is fed more than 1/4 pound.

Where to Source Green Tripe: I order green tripe (blended with ground trachea and gullet) through a local raw food co-op and bison tripe from Darwin's Pet. There are several brands that offer frozen and freeze-dried green tripe.

Canned Green Tripe: I no longer give our dogs canned green tripe because (1) it's cooked so our dogs don't get all of the nutrients, (2) some contain carrageenan gum, which has been tied to health issues in pets, and (3) it's more expensive than buying actual green tripe.

Guidelines of Raw Feeding

One mistake I made was being too dedicated to the various guidelines that I read about raw feeding. At first, I fed BARF model, then Prey Model. I over fed Sydney because I was following a raw food calculator and I didn't adjust the amount to meet her activity level.

When it comes to raw feeding, it's important to understand the basic guidelines and then adapt the diet to what our dogs need. The following are a couple of changes I made for my dogs:

- Instead of replacing meat with vegetables; I follow the 80% meat, 10% bone, 5% liver and offal (secreting organs). And I mix in pureed vegetables or fermented vegetables into our dogs' raw meals. Vegetables make up a small percentage of their diet. I only add more when one of my dogs needs to lose weight.

- Instead of sticking to the raw food calculator (2% for weight loss, 2.5% to maintain, 3% for an active dog), I adjusted the amount to meet each dog's needs.

As I became more confident in taking charge of my dogs' nutrition and diet, I was able to adjust their diets to meet their various needs at a moment's notice. It's not as complicated as it was when I first started feeding a raw diet.

Holistic Veterinarians and Raw Feeding

5 Things I've Learned About Holistic Veterinarians

1 – A holistic veterinarian can be an amazing resource for raw feeding.

I take my dogs to two holistic veterinarians in our area, Dr. Yearout and Dr. Rennert, and both have taught me a lot about raw feeding. Dr. Yearout helped me develop my veggie mix by telling me which vegetables he wanted to see me add to my dogs' diet. And Dr. Rennert knows a lot about Chinese Medicine and helps me decipher warming and cooling foods for my dogs.

When I take my dogs to the vet, diet is always part of the discussion because they both believe in natural healing and it's amazing the difference food can make in our dogs' diet. For instance, when Sydney had yeasty ears, I used the following to treat them naturally and her ears have remained yeast free:

- mist a 50/50 mixture of Braggs apple cider vinegar and water in her ear and let sit

- clean her ears with a soft tissue that is also misted with the above mixture

- massage coconut oil (natural anti-fungal, antibacterial, anti-viral) into her clean ear

- add kefir to her diet for three days

It worked!

2 – Holistic veterinarians are more expensive than traditional veterinarians; sometimes.

A vet visit used to cost me $40-$45; a holistic vet visit can run over $75 so I won't take my dogs to the holistic vet for something that I can treat at home. That is until I found my current veterinarians who own their own practices and can adjust their prices as they see fit, which has saved me money.

Although I love our holistic vets, I do have a traditional vet whom I trust, who understands that I feed raw, and who takes care of illnesses and minor injuries. For example, when Scout had a fever of unknown origin, taking him to an emergency vet and then a specialist was the better move. And I kept his holistic vets up to date on his condition and treatment.

3 – Holistic veterinarians follow Susan Thixton of TruthAboutPetFood.com.

It was a pleasant surprise to learn that one of our holistic veterinarians follows the blog TruthAboutPetFood.com. We catch up on what Susan Thixton has written about during our visits.

4 – Holistic veterinarian medicine may be covered by pet insurance.

One thing I looked for when shopping for pet insurance was coverage of alternative care: acupuncture, chiropractic adjustments, laser therapy, physical therapy, hydrotherapy, and more. Don't depend on the pet insurance company's website — call them to confirm that holistic vet care is part of their policy (or part of an add-on to your policy).

Pet insurance won't cover titer tests or blood work, however, it will cover alternative care after an illness or injury.

5 – Not all holistic vets are down with raw feeding.

Holistic veterinarians who work in traditional practices may not be pushing prescription pet food down your throat, but they won't jump up and down because you've chosen to feed your dog raw meat.

3 Ways to Find a Holistic Veterinarian

1 – Search Online

With online reviews, it's a lot easier to find a holistic vet. If you discover a vet with low stars (3 instead of 5) go through the reviews to make sure that there aren't any left by bitter ex-clients. Yelp allows businesses to respond to reviews — it's good reading.

2 – Search the AHVMA

The American Holistic Veterinary Medical Association (AHVMA) has a directory of holistic veterinarians. Keep in mind that the list isn't exhaustive; not all holistic vets are listed.

3 – Ask for a Referral

If you have connected with raw feeders in your area, ask them for a referral for a holistic veterinarian. What I like about this method is that I can ask someone about their experience instead of trying to figure out if an online review is genuine.

Introducing a Raw Fed Dog to a New Veterinarian

My dogs see two holistic vets who support raw feeding, so you'd think that the concern of introducing my raw fed dogs to a new veterinarian would be in my past.

Well, it's not.

In September 2015, I was making breakfast for the dogs. Scout isn't a morning dog, but I slept late that day so he should have been up and ready to eat, he wasn't. Scout was listless and warm, so I took his temperature. It was at 105 degrees, which required a trip to the emergency vet.

When my dog was sick, I didn't care what the vets thought about the fact that I fed him a raw food diet. It did cross my mind that they may blame the diet for his illness. Thankfully the vet who treated Scout and the specialist who took over the case were familiar with raw feeding. Although they weren't proponents of the diet, they respected that it was a choice that many dog owners were making and other than Scout's fever, he was a healthy dog with a gorgeous coat and white/shiny teeth.

Four days later, Scout was on the mend after a round of antibiotics and anti-nausea drugs.

Introducing My Raw Fed Dogs to a Vet

The situation I described was urgent. Most of the time, we're trying to find a good vet and not everyone has access to a pro-raw, holistic veterinarian. In that case, here are the things that have helped me find a vet that was open to my choice to feed a raw diet and subjecting my dogs to minimal vaccinations.

1 – An In-Person Interview with the Vet

It may sound nuts, but I made an appointment with vets in our area and during our visit I let them know that I feed a raw diet, I believe in minimal vaccinations, and I like to understand my dog's health, so I ask a lot of questions and do a lot of research.

An in-person chat is the best because you can see the vet cringe when you say, "raw feeding," and "minimal vaccinations." And they can see that you're as serious as a heart attack and won't be swayed.

If the vet is open to hearing me out, I can explain the work I've done to learn how to take charge of my dogs' diet, what I feed to my dogs and why, where I source the ingredients and more.

2 – Show Off Your Knowledge

In my experience with veterinarians who aren't on board with raw feeding, one of their biggest concerns about feeding raw dog food is that we won't feed a balanced diet. So prove that you do feed a balanced diet. Share the veterinarians you follow, the magazines you read, and be prepared to answer a lot of questions.

- **Why don't you add cornmeal for energy?** – Because protein is a superior source of energy.

- **Dogs have evolved to eat grains.** – I agree. However, I don't believe that grains are species appropriate or healthy for my dogs.

- **You have to be careful about the bacteria.** – I agree, which is why I wash my hands, keep my kitchen clean, wash my dog's dishes, and practice other sanitary habits just as if I were making a chicken dinner for my family.

- **The bacteria can be harmful to your dogs.** – That's what I thought at first. However, I learned about the anatomy of dogs. They have antibacterial enzymes in their saliva and a shorter digestive tract that processes food quickly, keeping any remaining bacteria from setting up shop.

- **I hope you're worming your dogs regularly.** – Thankfully, with the exception of green tripe, my dogs eat human grade proteins, and there are no parasites in their meat. Plus everything arrives frozen from reputable sources.

- **You have to be careful with raw bones.** – Absolutely! When my dogs enjoy recreational and raw meaty bones, they do so under supervision. I choose bones that they can enjoy safely — beef knuckle bones, beef knee caps, duck necks, lamb necks, duck frames, and duck wings.

- **A raw diet isn't balanced.** – Each meal I feed to my dogs may not be balanced, but neither is each meal that I eat. I focus on balancing our dogs' diet over time, planning their meals and supplements to make sure they get everything they need nutritionally.

- **There's no proof that raw feeding is beneficial for dogs.** – There are no studies funded by pet food companies, however, if you do a little digging, you'll find several studies from around the world that show that fresh food is better than processed food. I'll be happy to send you the links.

This is an example of some of the questions I receive and answer. Think of the questions you've received, the arguments against raw feeding, and develop confident, well thought out responses. While there are vets who are aggressively anti-raw feeding, there are many who will support their clients if they are assured that we're going to do the work it takes to feed a balanced diet.

3 – Don't Mention Blogs to a Vet

Unless a vet is open to social media and blogs, mentioning that a blog is your resource isn't always a great idea. Many traditional vets that I've met immediately shut down when you mention Dr. Google and blogs as if researching dog nutrition makes us morons.

While you and I may know of many blogs and bloggers who are sharing correct information about dog nutrition, there are many people who are sharing inaccurate information that is sending dogs to the vet. When the only raw fed dogs that a vet sees are the ones that are victims of an unbalanced, poorly researched diet, then I can't blame them for not being on board with raw feeding.

4 – Proof is in Four Paws

And finally, allow a veterinarian to examine your dog. I was able to change a vet's mind in under 20 minutes. She started the exam with "you have to be careful with that" after we told her about our dogs' diet. 20 minutes later, she admitted that we had healthy dogs and wanted to know more about what we fed them and even offered some suggestions.

That experience taught me that just because a vet isn't promoting a raw food diet doesn't mean that they're anti-raw.

Meeting a new vet doesn't have to be a negative experience. With each interaction, I learned something new. And if a veterinarian isn't a good fit, then I moved on to the next.

Joint Health, Canine Arthritis, and Raw Feeding

My Dogs' Joint Health History

Rodrigo and Sydney developed joint issues early in life. I was told that it was because they were mixed breed, rescue dogs. I have explored several things that may have contributed to my dogs developing joint issues at such an early age.

- They were fed a kibble diet for large breed dogs; a food meant for Great Danes and Mastiffs, not Blue Heeler mixes.

- They were spayed and neutered at six months old, which some people believe is too young and can lead to joint health issues due to the lack of sex hormones needed to promote proper growth and maturity.

- They were subjected to annual vaccinations for the first two years of their lives which negatively impacted their immune system and growth.

- They were exposed to chemical flea and tick treatments for the first two years of their lives which negatively taxed their immune system.

It could be all of these reasons, a combination of these reasons, or none of these reasons. Scout and Zoey have been raw fed since they were six weeks old, they've never been exposed to chemical flea and tick repellents, and they've been subjected to minimal vaccinations. They haven't had any health issues beyond Scout's fever in 2015.

Regardless of why Rodrigo and Sydney developed joint issues, at some point, I had to stop living in the past and focus on how to treat my dogs today, and I'm happy to say that I've found a regimen that works for both of my dogs.

Rodrigo and Sydney – 7 Years Old

Rodrigo's and Sydney's joint issues began to resolve with a diet change. However, a partial cruciate tear brought about by Sydney's love of zoomies slowed her down. Her veterinarian said that surgery wasn't necessary and I allowed her to heal naturally. I made one mistake with Sydney; I didn't adjust how much I was feeding her. I thought that she wouldn't gain weight because she was on a raw diet. Yes, I know that I should have known better.

Rodrigo and Sydney were transitioned to raw in 2013 and their joint health has improved due to:

- Feeding a balanced raw diet is important. A kibble diet, filled with grains and starch, is highly inflammatory. However, a balanced raw diet gives my dogs everything they needs to build strong muscles to support their joints and bones. And their joints are no longer carrying the extra weight they gained on a kibble diet.

- I add fish oil, sardines, and salmon to my dog's diet. Fish oil and fish offer anti-inflammatory properties to promote improved joint health.

- I add 1-1/2 teaspoons of golden paste to each of their meals five days a week. I began using golden paste for the pain relief, but it's also great or digestive health, and it's said that it can prevent the growth of tumors. My dogs aren't fans of the taste of golden paste alone but they don't seem to notice it when I add it to their raw meals.

- I feed my dogs duck feet, beef trachea, emu cartilage, bone broth, and other foods that are rich in glucosamine and chondroitin and promote joint health.

- My dogs exercise daily. While Rodrigo is more active, Sydney is a bit slower and she and I walk around our property together daily.

On the rare occasions when one of my dogs exhibits joint pain, I'll give him/her an anti-inflammatory recommended by their vet with CBD oil for pets before bedtime.

Works every time.

Avoiding Inflammation by Feeding Fresh Food

Because I'm 100% responsible for my dogs' diet, I'm very careful about which foods I add to the rotation. I never add raw chicken to my dogs' diet because I'm concerned about the sourcing and the over exposure of this protein in our dogs' diet. If you visit your local pet store and review ingredients in food and treats, you'll find chicken, chicken, and more chicken. I think this protein has become an inflammatory for our dogs, leading to allergies and joint issues. So no raw chicken.

Thanks to my co-op, I have access to many proteins and when adding something new to their diet, I go slowly until I see how my dogs react before adding the new protein as a staple to their diet. Guinea hen and alpaca have worked out great for three of my dogs, but not for Rodrigo.

And while some foods are high in Omega 6 fatty acids, which contributes to inflammation, they can be offset by feeding foods high in Omega 3 fatty acids (organ meat, sardines, salmon, mackerel) to offset the Omega 6s.

Rodrigo and Sydney are officially senior dogs now, but they're still happy, active (Rodrigo more so than Sydney) dogs and I have the raw food diet to thank. A friend recently celebrated his dog's 18th birthday; he feeds raw too. When he told me, I was overjoyed, because I can look forward to many more years with Rigo and Syd-Syd.

Knowledge, Kicked Out, Kibble, and Raw Feeding

Sharing Your Knowledge About Raw Feeding

When it comes to raw feeding unless you feed a 100% premade raw diet or have someone who can work with you, homework will be required. I read books, I grilled many veterinarians with questions, I followed leaders in the raw feeding community, and I joined Facebook groups. All of these resources helped me grow from a person who was worried that she'd harm her dogs to someone who makes raw food while binge-watching television.

I changed the focus of Keep the Tail Wagging® to raw feeding and dog nutrition when I realized how hard it is to learn how to feed our dogs. Over the years, I've learned a few things about sharing what I learn about raw feeding with others.

- **I don't push my knowledge on to others.** If a Facebook friend shares a picture a bag of kibble, I don't send a private message or leave a comment critiquing their choices in dog food and recommending raw. From personal experience, it's better to ask people if they're interested in your thoughts than push your thoughts on them.

- **Don't assume that people feed kibble out of ignorance.** There are many reasons why someone won't home cook or feed raw to their dogs. Someone's dog may not be able to eat raw due to a compromised immune system (human or dog) and may be concerned about safety. Someone may not have access to raw ingredients or premade raw. Or someone may not have the time to put into learning about raw feeding and switching to the diet.

- **Don't hate on people for not feeding raw.** I see this daily in Facebook groups, people judging friends, family members, and strangers for feeding kibble. I will admit that I have judged people as well, but then I take a step back and remind myself that five years ago, I thought I was doing great by feeding a quality kibble.

- **Be open to other perspectives.** I recently received an email from someone who told me that she didn't like my Facebook raw feeding group because she was trying to educate us and we were sharing different opinions, which made her feel attacked. I was disappointed to see her go, but I agree that my Facebook group wasn't the group for her because it was created to allow people from all around the world, with varying levels of experience, to share what they're learning. The discussions we're having are amazing and I've made many beneficial changes to my dogs' diet because people have shared what they're doing.

- **Continue sharing content about the benefits of raw feeding.** While it may seem like no one is listening, one day a friend will have a question about dog nutrition and you'll be their resource because you're always sharing articles and blog posts on the topic.

If you want to share your knowledge about raw feeding with others, do so gently, respectfully, and without expecting people to change. It took me six months to start making plans to transition my dogs to raw because I wanted to make sure I knew what I was doing. Be patient and be kind.

Being Kicked Out of a Raw Feeding Group

If you're an inquisitive person like me then you will be kicked out of a raw feeding group eventually. To make navigating the world of Facebook raw feeding groups easier, I offer the following suggestions:

- **Read the group rules/guidelines.** If the group says, "no kibble talk," don't ask people what kibble they recommend. If the group doesn't recommend vegetables, then don't share images of your dog's breakfast with broccoli, carrots, and kale. The guidelines are a great way to know what to expect and just because the rules are strict doesn't mean that you won't learn anything. Remember, there are loads of raw feeding groups on Facebook and if you're discouraged from eating vegetables in Group A, Group B may welcome the discussions.

- **Don't take disagreements personally.** There are going to be times when people question the choices you make for your dog's diet or offer advice that is contrary to what you shared when joining a discussion. Although it can feel like people aren't hearing you, don't take it personally. Unless someone prefaces their advice with "Hey! Moron!!!" then take everything as an opportunity to learn something new. And if you do feel attacked, don't engage. It's best to walk away from an aggressive discussion than engage with a rude person. It's pointless to argue with a troll or someone who is having a supremely crappy day. Walk away.

- **And if you're kicked out, move on.** It's tempting to crow to the world about the unfairness of being kicked out of a Facebook group. Only crow if you find it funny. The reason I started a raw feeding group called The Raw Feeders 'Kicked Out' Club is because I kept getting kicked out of raw feeding groups. It became such a joke that people would add me to groups just to ban me. I've been accused of joining groups to start trouble (I asked if it was okay to discuss vegetables), of joining a group to steal one of the Admin's content (because they saw that I share a lot of articles on raw feeding on Facebook), and of poisoning my dogs (because I follow the BARF model of raw feeding). I was offended at first, but each time I got the boot, I saw the humor in all of it.

Facebook raw feeding groups are a fantastic place to learn more about raw feeding, to connect with other raw feeders, and to chat with people who understand why you feed raw. Not every group is for every raw feeder; take your time and you'll find the group that is right for you and your dogs.

Feeding Kibble and Fresh Food

One of the biggest fears many raw feeders have is having to go back to feeding their dogs a kibble diet after they've learned what goes into processed dog food. However, I'm no longer convinced that it's the end of the world if I have to feed kibble (but I don't want to do it).

If I find myself in a position where raw feeding is no longer feasible, I will do the following to improve the quality of the kibble I feed to my dogs:

- **I will feed Carna4 because it's the best.** Kibble isn't ideal and not something I want to feed to my dogs due to the excessive processing, mystery ingredients, and questionable sourcing. Carna4 has minimal ingredients, no synthetic vitamins, and it's slow baked and minimally processed.

- **I will soak the kibble in bone broth.** Bone broth is a nutritious food that I give to my dogs as a treat, when they have an upset tummy or low appetite, and to help boost joint and immune system health. Soaking kibble in bone broth will make it easier for dogs to digest while pumping natural, fresh nutrients into their system.

- **I will add fresh food to my dogs' meals.** I have a glorious pressure cooker that makes it easy to mix up a cooked meal for my dogs that I can add to my dogs' meals as a food topper. I'd also add sardines, green lipped mussels, and give my dogs a treat of raw goat milk, Ewegurt, or fermented fish stock.

- **I will keep fresh water available.** Dry dog food is “dry” and if a dog isn't properly hydrated, a diet of dry dog food will leave them in a state of perpetual dehydration. Therefore, I will keep plenty of fresh water (keeping their dishes clean) available to keep them hydrated.

Liver, Liver Health, and Raw Feeding

Feeding Liver to My Dogs

The other day I received an email from someone asking me if they should add liver to their dog's raw diet. The person was unknowingly feeding an unbalanced raw diet and she thought adding liver would add more nutrients. She was right and wrong and I received a heavy dose of Déjà vu.

I remember trying to understand the ins and outs of raw feeding and it wasn't easy. I learned early on that feeding liver can be tricky.

5% of my dogs' raw diet is liver, which I expand upon below. Although I've fed turkey, pork, and venison liver, today, I primarily feed an organ/tripe blend from GreenTripe.com. And I cook chicken or beef liver for the dogs as a food topper or treat few times a year.

WHY IT'S IMPORTANT TO FEED LIVER TO OUR DOGS

- The liver is loaded with nutrients and in a raw diet that follows the 80/10/10 rule (80% muscle meat, 10% bone, and 10% organ), liver serves as 5% of the ingredients. In other words, the 10% = 5% offal (secreting organs like kidneys, spleen, pancreas) and 5% liver.

- Feeding liver also supports liver health. However, if your dog has copper storage hepatopathy or abnormal accumulation of copper, feeding liver can be tricky. I've been told by veterinarians that feeding too much liver can negatively affect the liver of healthy dogs. Speak to your holistic vet about supporting your dog's liver health through diet.

- The liver is rich and will cause diarrhea if too much is fed. When adding it to a puppy's diet and the raw diet of a dog new to raw feeding, it's important to start small and build up. I've learned to start puppies and small dogs at 1/3 teaspoon and start larger dogs at 1/2 teaspoon; working up to 5% of their diet.

- A liver's job is to clear all the toxins from an animal's system. Some people have warned me that some liver from wild game can make my dogs sick due to the toxins. Others have shared that the liver filters toxins out; it doesn't hoard them in the system. So, to be safe, I feed my dogs human grade liver.

GreenTripe.com

I order food by the case from GreenTripe.com through our local raw food co-op. My regular orders include:

- Green Tripe / Trachea / Gullet blend – I feed 2-3 meals per week.

- Green Tripe / Organ blend – I add this to my dogs' raw meals to account for the organ/offal. It contains beef heart, lungs, liver, spleen, and pancreas with green tripe. This is the only source of lungs, spleen, and pancreas I've found.

- Xkaliber blend, which is great for highly active dogs and seniors and contains green tripe, muscle meat, heart, tongue, trachea/gullet and ground Bone – I feed 1 meal per week to Scout, who is our most active dog.

The only disappointment of using GreenTripe.com's organ blend is that they don't offer the percentages of the mix and because it contains heart, I know that it's not 5% offal, 5% liver — adding the muscle meat throws that percentage off. I do trust this brand, however, I occasionally add a small amount of liver and kidney to my dogs' raw diet in an attempt to balance out the organ meat over time.

Models of Raw Feeding for Dogs

Models of Raw Feeding

When you join the raw feeding community, it doesn't take long for you to realize that no one feeds raw the same way. Over the past four years, I've fed premade raw, BARF Model, FrankenPrey Model and today, I feed a model I lovingly call FrankenBARF.

The pros and cons of each diet that I list below are based on my experience. Not all raw feeders will agree.

Premade Raw Dog Food

So premade raw isn't considered a "model" of raw feeding, but with the growth of the raw sector over the past couple of years, I think it deserves mention. Premade Raw Dog Food is commercial raw that you buy at the pet store, order online, or buy directly from brands. I've fed many premade raw brands, however, as I began learning more about dog nutrition, I realized that making raw food at home food is my best option.

BENEFITS OF FEEDING PREMADE RAW

- We don't have to worry about balancing the diet.
- Access to more proteins.
- No need to buy extra freezers to store bulk orders, unless you have a lot of big dogs.
- It's quick and easy to feed with little mess; plus it can be fed in a dog dish.

DOWNSIDES OF FEEDING PREMADE RAW

- Some premade raw brands use HPP (high-pressure pasteurization) processing to kill off bacteria; while this makes raw feeding an option for more people — my opinion is that the processing kills off important nutrients requiring more supplementation.

- Feeding premade raw is expensive because the brand takes care of sourcing and balancing for you.

- Some premade raw brands use synthetic vitamins to make the diet balanced.

- Some premade raw brands try to attain balance based on AAFCO standards, which were created for a kibble/canned diet — not a raw food diet.

BARF Model Raw Feeding

BARF ('biologically appropriate raw food' or 'bones and raw food') model raw feeding includes:

- 65%-75% muscle meat
- 10%-15% bone
- 5% liver
- 5% offal (secreting organs like kidney and spleen)
- 5%-10% fruits, vegetables, dairy

If you search ratios for BARF model, you'll find several ranges with muscle meat being as low as 45% and bone content as high as 50%. BARF model also encourages supplementation when needed.

BENEFITS OF FEEDING BARF MODEL

- Dogs have more access to nutrients with the addition of vegetables, fruit, dairy, and supplements.

- Easier to meat your dog's needs because supplements are acceptable.

- Ground raw dog food is acceptable and easier to feed.

- Raw meaty bones and recreational bones are added separately for teeth cleaning.

DOWNSIDES TO FEEDING BARF MODEL

- Dogs eat faster because ground raw is easier to gulp.

- Ground raw doesn't offer the teeth cleaning benefits of eating whole raw.

- To make raw feeding more affordable, you may have to invest in additional freezers to store bulk purchases.

- Vegetables need to be pureed to help dogs absorb the nutrients.

- Some dogs won't eat vegetables.

Prey Model Raw Feeding

- 80% muscle meat

- 10% bone

- 5% liver

- 5% offal (secreting organs like kidney and spleen)

The Prey model discourages the use of vegetables, fruit, and over supplementation. In the Prey Model, dogs can get everything they need through diet. For example, instead of fish oil, feed sardines and mackerel. Instead of a digestive supplement, trust the living enzymes in raw food and add green tripe.

BENEFITS OF FEEDING PREY MODEL

- Dogs are eating in a way that is more reminiscent of wolves.

- Whole raw allows dogs to satisfy their chew drive, clean their teeth, and work their jaw and shoulder muscles.

- Dogs take longer to finish their meal, which is great for their digestive system.

DOWNSIDES TO FEEDING PREY MODEL

- To make raw feeding more affordable, you may have to invest in additional freezers to store bulk purchases.

- Ground raw dog food isn't always acceptable in this model.

- Feeding whole raw can be challenging for some people/dogs because some dogs need to be taught to eat whole raw (and not gulp) and to eat on a tarp if fed indoors.

FrankenBARF Model Raw Feeding

FrankenBARF model raw feeding includes:

- 80% muscle meat

- 10% bone

- 5% liver

- 5% offal (secreting organs like kidney and spleen)

Vegetables, goats milk, raw eggs, supplements — all added in addition to the above to provide additional nutrients and satisfy each dog's specific needs.

BENEFITS OF FEEDING FRANKENBARF MODEL

- It's easier to meet the needs of each of my dogs when I modify the BARF model.

- Dogs have more access to nutrients with the addition of vegetables, dairy, and supplements.

- Easier to balance a raw diet because supplements are acceptable.

- Ground raw dog food is acceptable and easier to feed. However, whole raw is fed too, satisfying a dog's chew drive and cleaning their teeth.

- Raw meaty bones and recreational bones are added separately for teeth cleaning.

DOWNSIDES TO FEEDING FRANKENBARF MODEL

- A lot of time goes into grinding meat and mixing ingredients; a quality meat grinder is a must if you plan to feed ground raw.

- To make raw feeding more affordable, you may have to invest in additional freezers to store bulk purchases.

- Vegetables need to be pureed to help dogs absorb the nutrients.

The Prey model can also be adapted and fed as FrankenPrey; this isn't something that I've tried with my dogs, however, I know many people who feed a customized version of Prey model.

Choosing the Right Model for Your Dog

Learning how to feed my dogs is all about trial and error. This year, four years after I started feeding raw, each of my dogs are finally eating a diet that is tailored to their individual needs. However, I'm always learning about ingredients, supplements, and practices that may provide more benefits. For example…

- Some people fast their dog one day a week; I allow my dogs to self-fast.

- I began adding dehydrated mushrooms to my vegetable mix.

- I now consistently feed my dogs eggs 3 days a week.

- I replaced digestive supplements with fermented foods.

I recommend considering all models when you're new to raw feeding and be prepared to make adjustments when necessary.

Natural Vitamins, New Proteins, and Raw Feeding

Natural Vitamins and Raw Feeding

During my first year of raw feeding, I ordered tons of supplements from Amazon – I didn't understand about synthetic vitamins, sourcing, or that raw fed dogs absorbed nutrients and living enzymes from the meat and bone in their diet. While I do buy supplements when I can't find a natural source, I'm more particular about what I give to my dogs.

The below table offer sources of various vitamins and minerals. This is not an exhaustive list.

Vitamin A: skin, vision, immune system — raw eggs, liver, spinach, kale, broccoli, carrots, greens, pumpkin

Vitamin B: overall growth of our dogs — spirulina, raw goat milk, kefir

Vitamin C: immune system — kale, broccoli

Vitamin D: regulates calcium and phosphorous levels — fatty fish, raw goat milk, liver, beef

Vitamin E: cell function, fat metabolism, anti-oxidant — liver, kale, spinach, greens, broccoli, parsley

Vitamin K: healthy blood functions — kale, cabbage, broccoli, kefir, asparagus

Calcium:Phosphorous: strong teeth and bones, supports heart, muscle, and never functions — green tripe, egg shells

Iron: blood health, energy, immune system — red meat, liver, eggs

Magnesium: healthy bones, muscles, nerve systems, enzyme functions —

spinach, broccoli, green beans

While my dogs get most of their vitamins and minerals through their raw diet, I do add various supplements to make sure my dogs get what they need.

- Spirulina (helps with immune system health)
- LifeLine Ocean Kelp (helps with metabolism health)
- Fish Oil (benefits joints and skin and coat health)
- Milk Thistle (helps to support liver health and naturally detoxes the system)

While it seems like we need to scramble to make sure our dogs are getting all of these vitamins, it's really not necessary. I don't give the vitamins much thought beyond alternating the supplements I listed above and making sure my dogs get a raw egg at least three times a week (personal preference, not something someone told me to do). My dogs get everything else through their raw diet.

Raw feeding is trial and error. The longer I follow leaders in this community, read articles, and attend online webinars, the more changes I see. While it's tempting to drop everything I'm doing and make changes according to new science, it's not a good idea. Instead, I'm going to do what's working for my dogs and if new science provides the answer to a current problem or clarifies something, then I'll slowly incorporate changes.

New Proteins and Raw Feeding

One of the things I love about raw feeding is the ability to easily expose my dogs to new proteins. Rodrigo has an intolerance to several proteins. I had him tested several years ago through a local nutritionist and I learned that my dog cannot eat to chicken, turkey, beef, salmon, lamb, and peas.

Today, he still cannot eat chicken, turkey, and beef; but he can eat green beef tripe, salmon, and lamb. I don't feed my dogs peas so that's a non-issue.

At first, Rodrigo's protein intolerance limited what I could feed him, but with raw feeding and access to amazing sources including our raw food co-op, we have a lot of options:

- Duck
- Pork
- Rabbit
- Pheasant and Quail (Columbia River)
- Lamb (Darwin's Pet or NW Naturals)
- Venison, Elk, and Bison
- Sardines and Mackerel
- Goat and Smelt (Raw Paws Pet Food)

I've learned to buy small amounts when I can and if I can't, then I have three other dogs who can eat the food and local raw feeding friends who are happy to swap food with me.

Organ Meat, Offal, and Raw Feeding

Organ Meat vs. Offal in Raw Feeding

Despite spending a year researching raw dog food, I honestly thought that I just needed to add liver to my dogs' diet. Not only was this wrong, my dogs got diarrhea because I fed too much liver because I thought I could eyeball their meal and figure out the 80/10/5/5 by sight.

Yep, I made many mistakes.

I feed my dogs a modified version of the BARF (biologically appropriate raw food) Model. When I was comparing BARF to Prey Model, I came to the conclusion that I wasn't okay with taking away muscle meat or increasing bone to incorporate vegetables. So I created a model that works for my dogs - FrankenBARF.

- 80% muscle meat
- 10% bone
- 5% liver
- 5% offal (secreting organs)
- vegetables, dairy, eggs, and supplements

When it comes to making raw dog food some of the meats that we as humans identify as "organ meat" fall into the muscle meat column.

Organs Fed as Muscle Meat	Organs Fed as Offal	Other Cuts of Meat Fed as Muscle
Heart	Pancreas	Green Tripe
Gizzard	Kidney	Trachea

Lung	Spleen	Tongue
	Testicles	
	Brain	

Why We Feed Offal to Dogs

Organ meat (offal) is packed with nutrients and the least expensive part of my dogs' diet, so they never go without.

- Vitamins: A, B, D, E, and K
- Minerals: calcium, phosphorus, magnesium, manganese, iron, copper, iodine, potassium, sodium, selenium, and zinc
- Omega-3 fats EPA and DHA

QUALITY SOURCES FOR OFFAL

I thought the easiest source for offal was the local grocery store; I was wrong. Our store only carries liver. I've heard that you can get variety at an Asian Market, but I have yet to explore one thoroughly. So I order all of my ingredients through a local raw food co-op.

- pork kidneys
- pancreas
- green tripe/organ blend that contains liver, spleen, and pancreas*
- organ blend with liver and kidney*
- venison, pork, or turkey liver

** With the organ blends on the market (sold by GreenTripe.com and Columbia River Pet Foods) request the amount of each ingredient. If an amount isn't available, then look at the order of the ingredients with the theory that the first ingredient is the most; the last is the least.*

HOW I FEED OFFAL TO MY DOGS

My dogs eat a partially ground raw food diet. Usually, I grind pork kidneys, turkey liver (because it's small), and mix it with an organ blend that contains pancreas and spleen.

HOW MUCH OFFAL I FEED TO MY DOGS

Offal is 10% of my dogs' raw diet, and half of that 5% is liver. I started low and worked my way up because organ meat is rich. To decide how much offal to add to my raw dog food, I do the following calculation:

Step One: calculate the bone

- 40 pounds of duck wings = 61% muscle meat and 39% bone
- 40 pounds of duck wings x 39% = 15.6 pounds of bone

Step Two: calculate the offal (this is easy)

- 15.6 pounds / 2 = 7.8 pounds of offal and 7.8 pounds of liver

Step Three: calculate the total amount of muscle, offal, and bone

- 15.60 pounds of bone / 10% = 156 pounds of total meat (muscle, offal, and bone)

Step Four: calculate the additional muscle meat needed

- 156 pounds x 80% = 124.8 pounds less 24.4 pounds (this is 61% of the duck wings) = 100.4 pounds of muscle meat
- To make up the 100.4 pounds, I add trim (muscle meat, no bones), gizzards, and hearts

Step Five: mix everything together and freeze

- I usually make seven days of meals every other week. I alternate this food with other proteins to provide variety: duck, venison, emu, rabbit, green beef tripe.

It's important to note that although this calculation appeases the number crunchers in the world (I'm one of them), it's not necessary. I found that it's easier to balance a dog's raw diet over time instead of within each meal.

WHAT IF MY DOG WON'T EAT ORGAN MEAT

Some dogs don't like the texture of organ meat, for these dogs, you can try the following:

- If the organ meat is whole, try grinding it and mixing it into a raw blend.

- Slightly cook organ meat, cooking it less over time until your dog acclimates to the texture.

- Feed freeze-dried organ meat.

Pork, Parasites, Pancreas, and Raw Feeding

Feeding Pork in a Raw Food Diet

For the longest time, I would only feed pork if it came from a premade brand – Answers Pet Food, Steve's Real Food, or Vital Essentials Raw. I was worried about trichinosis and other parasites making my dogs sick. After more experience and research, I learned that I didn't have to worry if I was buying my proteins from a quality source because trichinosis was eradicated in the US food system a long time ago. Today, I buy human-grade pork products — kidneys, liver, hearts — and placed my first order for pork cushion meat in 2017.

I love the idea of adding pork back into my dogs' diet. And although I would love to continue feeding premade, I can mix up raw dog food using human-grade pork products for less.

PARASITES AND RAW FEEDING

Another fear people have of raw feeding is bacteria and parasites. Dogs are equipped to handle bacteria due to an enzyme in their saliva that kills bacteria, a highly acidic gut that makes it difficult for bacteria to thrive, and a shorter digestive tract equipped to absorb nutrients and push food through quickly.

BUT WHAT ABOUT PARASITES?

The only food in my freezers that come with a risk of parasites are wild game and raw fish. I rarely feed either, however, when I do, I freeze everything for at least a month (many people recommend 1-2 weeks).

The lack of raw fish and wild game in my dogs' diet doesn't protect them from parasites when they kill and dine on small animals on our property. When I find the remains of a woodland creature, the dogs go through a parasite treatment: 1 tablespoon of food grade diatomaceous earth per day for

7 days.

Diatomaceous earth (DE) is a white powder that is derived from the fossilized remains of marine phytoplankton. When it comes into contact with parasites, it dehydrates their bodies, killing them so they pass through a dog's digestive system in the stool. I was recently told that once DE is introduced to a damp environment (our digestive system), it is no longer effective. For me, the jury is still out on that theory because I've found more information supporting the use of diatomaceous earth through diet.

Pancreas and Raw Feeding

This year I diagnosed Rodrigo with EPI. I know we shouldn't diagnose via Google, however, this time, it worked. I was doing some homework on feeding pancreas when I discovered a condition called Exocrine Pancreatic Insufficiency (EPI) where the pancreas isn't producing enough digestive enzymes in a dog's gut.

SYMPTOMS OF EPI INCLUDE:

- Continued weight loss despite always being hungry
- Pooping more often than the other dogs; poop is larger, yellow or gray in color, and soft
- Dog eats his own poop (coprophagia)
- Increased gas and tummy noises
- Occasional diarrhea and vomiting
- Increased anxiety, fearful behavior

A veterinarian can conduct a test to confirm EPI, but I chose to save the clinic fee and start Rodrigo on a pancreas supplement I discovered that's helping dogs and cats with EPI or EPI-like symptoms. I saw an immediate improvement in Rodrigo's health and behavior. Six months later, I introduced Rodrigo to fermented foods, decreasing dependence of the pancreas supplements, and continued to see improved gut health in my dog.

Transitioning to raw feeding cleared up most of Rodrigo's health issues (allergies, skin rashes, ear infections, itchy paws, joint pain). Although his gut issues improved, he still had bad weeks. Rodrigo hasn't had a bad week since I began adding the pancreas supplement, and subsequently, fermented foods to his diet.

- He's gained a little bit of weight
- His poop is smaller than it used to be and a normal color
- He no longer eats his poop
- He has a normal amount of gas
- No more diarrhea and loose stool
- His anxiety and aggressive have calmed greatly

Speaking with a holistic veterinarian about Rodrigo's medical history, symptoms, and behavior ruled out EPI. The reason Rodrigo isn't able to produce enough digestive enzymes is due to repeated rounds of antibiotics his first veterinarian prescribed to combat the symptoms of food intolerances and environmental allergies. This treatment ruined the stomach lining of Rodrigo's gut. The fermented foods I add to his diet provides the support he needs to digest the nutrients in his meals.

PANREAS SUPPLEMENT vs. RAW PANCREAS:

I want to try adding raw pancreas to his diet, however, it's a bit high maintenance:

- I've been advised to add 2 ounces of pancreas for every 20 pounds of body weight; Rodrigo would get 6 ounces twice a day.
- Feeding more than that is not recommended and can cause damage to the pancreas.
- To maximize enzyme efficiency, we need to whip pancreas with a fork or wire whisk to a pudding-like consistency or liquify in a

blender.

- Pancreas needs to be served at room temperature.

- Pancreas has a shelf life of only 3 months which I'll have to take into mind when ordering.

Although I have found a pancreas supplement for Rodrigo, I would like to try raw pancreas and plan to place an order through our co-op and invest in a dedicated blender.

FERMENTED FOODS FOR DOGS:

Adding fermented foods to my dogs' diet turned out to be better than pancreas or pancreas supplement for Rodrigo, or a digestive supplement for my other dogs:

- Fermented foods have a higher level of natural probiotics than supplements and are easier to feed than raw pancreas.

- Fermented foods improve gut and immune system health.

- Fermented foods serve to naturally detox our dogs' systems, further improving health.

- Fermented foods are generally found in the refrigerated section of natural grocery stores — look for brands that don't have onions and a low sodium percentage.

- There are many recipes to make fermented foods can be made at home with shredded vegetables and they don't require much salt. You can also choose to use a culture starter in lieu of salt.

I currently add 1 tbsp of fermented vegetables to each of our dog's raw meals four days per week.

Quality Brands, Questions, and Raw Feeding

Finding Quality Raw Dog Food Brands

Have you noticed that there are more brands entering the raw feeding market? I have a Google Alert set up to learn about new brands and it's exciting to see so many options available or dogs and cats. However, just because a brand makes raw dog food doesn't mean that we should feed it to our dogs.

Because of Rodrigo's digestive issues and protein allergies, I have to be careful about his diet. I've finally stopped exposing him to raw brands other than a small set and new brands are a No Go for him because I've come across many that add chicken to their recipes, use synthetic vitamins, and have proprietary (aka secret) recipes. I like to know the sourcing and the ingredients before I feed a food to my dogs.

Of course, every dog is different and what doesn't work for Rodrigo may work great for my other dogs or your dogs. Below is a list of quality raw food brands that I trust and will feed to my dogs.

- Darwin's Pet – lamb, green bison tripe
- GreenTripe.com – green beef tripe
- Vital Essentials Raw – wild boar
- Answers Pet Food – pork
- Steve's Real Food – pork
- Columbia River Pet Food – guinea hen (for the girls only), quail, pheasant
- Raw Paws Pet Food – goat and smelt

- NW Naturals - white fish and salmon, lamb

The reason these brands made the list is because their customer service is amazing, my dogs do well on their food, and I can buy most of them through our local co-op. Darwin's Pet isn't available through the co-op, therefore, I have a recurring order with Darwin's.

There are tons of quality brands available for dogs and cats. At the moment, I feed a limited amount of premade raw dog food because it can be expensive. The exception is lamb, which took me by surprise. Lamb is expensive in my area and it's more affordable for me to buy it premade from Darwin's or NW Naturals.

Questions About Raw Feeding

I began feeding raw in April 2013. At that time, I thought a day would come when I would know it all — that day will never come. I will always have questions about raw feeding. My questions go from the mundane — if Dr. Barbara Royal is Oprah's veterinarian, does that mean Oprah is a raw feeder? — to the complicated — is it possible for my dogs to have a thyroid condition despite the fact that she tested negative for hypothyroidism?

Although the raw feeding learning curve isn't as steep as it was several years ago, I still have a lot to learn and I will always have questions and the following helps:

- It's good to have a holistic vet (or two) who is experienced in raw feeding.

- Join a friendly raw feeding group that is open to answering questions and exploring all aspects of raw feeding.

- Look for opportunities to learn more — books, webinars, seminars, workshops.

- And network with other local raw feeders to share experiences and tips.

When it comes to raw feeding, I'm surprised by how many questions I have — both random and complicated. We never stop learning.

Recreational Bones, Raw Meaty Bones, and Raw Feeding

Feeding My Dogs Raw Bones

When I began feeding my dogs a raw diet, I knew that raw bones were part of the regime, but I was nervous because…

- raw bones can break teeth
- raw bones can splinter and cause injury
- raw bones can create a blockage

It took me a while to become comfortable with feeding raw bones to my dogs. One day, I decided to allow my Control-Freak Flag to fly and I allowed my dogs to try various bones; a new one each weekend. This taught me the bones that weren't a good fit for them and the ones that were safe.

Finding Safe Raw Bones for Dogs

I always supervise my dogs when they're eating their raw bones. If they look like they're about to swallow a bone whole, if a bone starts splintering, or if Rodrigo decides to steal everyone's bones – I can step in before we have a situation.

After a few weeks of testing out bones, I found four raw meaty bones and three recreational bones that worked out great for my dogs.

RAW BONES THAT WORK WITH MY DOGS

Raw Meaty Bones	Recreational Bones
Duck Necks	Beef Knuckle Bones

Lamb Necks	Beef Knee Caps
Turkey Necks	Buffalo Knuckle Bones
Duck Frames	

Benefits of Feeding Raw Bones to Dogs

While there are several health benefits to feeding raw bones to dogs, I'll be honest and admit that I give them to my dogs to get a block of peace and quiet in a house with four dogs. A raw bone keeps the dogs still, quiet, and focused on their chewing. I can work on my blog, read a book, or just enjoy a nice afternoon. I only give our dogs raw bones in the spring and summer on nice days because they eat them outside.

Since this isn't all about me, let me share other reasons raw bones are good for my dogs.

- Cleans their teeth and gums.
- Helps to strengthen their jaw, neck, and shoulder muscles.
- Satisfies their chew drive.
- And, in the case of raw meaty bones, provides a small meal.

Alternatives to Raw Bones for Dogs

As I mentioned, I feed my dogs raw bones outside. In the winter, it's too cold to supervise their bone chewing outside and my boyfriend isn't comfortable with me laying tarps around the house for inside enjoyment. What sucks is that by the time spring and summer roll around, my dogs have a little plaque buildup. So I have a few alternatives.

- Bully sticks
- Cold smoked bones

- Dehydrated beef trachea, gullet
- Dehydrated duck feet, chicken feet, turkey feet
- Himalayan chews

The alternatives we give to our dogs keep the plaque down and occupy our dogs while satisfying their chew drive, but not as well as raw bones.

Supplements and Raw Feeding

Why I Add Supplements to My Dogs' Diet

I feed my dogs a modified raw diet based on the BARF (biologically appropriate raw food) model. I call it FrankenBARF and it is:

- 80% muscle meat
- 10% bone
- 5% liver
- 5% offal (secreting organs)
- organic vegetables, dairy, eggs, oceanic kelp, and supplements

My goal is to provide my dogs with the nutrients they need and I don't think that this is possible with a diet of raw meat and bone alone for Rodrigo and Sydney. Both of my older dogs have health issues that have since been cleared up on a raw food diet. Scout and Zoey, who have been raw fed since they were 6 weeks old, receive very little supplementation to their diet.

SUPPLEMENTS I ADD TO MY DOGS' DIET AND WHY

I don't add supplements daily (although that's how I started). It's not necessary because my dogs get so much from their raw diet. However, the supplements add a much-needed health boost and today, I supplement my dogs' meals 4 days a week (depending on the supplement and the dog).

Digestive Supplement: After several years of trying various digestive supplements, probiotics, and prebiotics, I settled on adding fermented foods (vegetables, fish stock, and kefir) to my dogs' diet several times a week to support their digestive health.

Fish Oil: I add fish oil to my dogs' diet because the Omega 3 fatty acids help with skin and coat health, brain development, allergies, joint health, digestive health, and more while offsetting the Omega 6 fatty acids in meat. I also add sardines, mackerel, and salmon when it's available.

Joint Supplement: I replaced the joint supplements I used for whole foods that are naturally high in glucosamine and chondroitin for joint support. The food they prefer are duck feet and beef trachea. And I add bone broth (made from joint bones) or fermented fish stock to their raw meals several times a week.

Turmeric Paste aka Golden Paste: Rodrigo developed arthritis before he turned two. Sydney shortly after. Feeding a raw diet reduced inflammation, but didn't completely eliminate the pain. Sydney also had a partial tear to her left, rear cruciate that healed naturally. The golden paste has done wonders for my dogs and they are active and happy today.

Canine System Saver (Sydney): This is an all-natural supplement that I was introduced to a couple of years ago and I love it. I add CSS to Sydney's meals each morning and the improvement in her mobility has been amazing; she's playful, active, and a little bit naughty. This supplement is truly amazing.

Spirulina: I began adding spirulina to my dogs' diet to curb the grass eating habit. A nutritionist told me that dogs eat grass when they have an upset stomach and when they are looking for a nutrient found in spirulina. A small amount goes a long way with this one and I only add it a few days a week.

Milk Thistle: I add milk thistle to Sydney's diet several days a week to boost her liver health, which, according to her veterinarian, is linked to her joint and ligament health. I also give the dogs a milk thistle detox three times a year, splitting one container between all the dogs for approximately 1-1/2 - 2 weeks.

Transitioning a Dog to Raw Feeding

3 Ways to Transition a Dog to Raw Feeding

Earlier in the book, I share steps to help you transition a dog to a raw food diet, however, that's not the only path.

When I began feeding a raw food diet, I didn't think I could switch straight away; I was in several raw feeding groups, receiving contradictory information. So I returned to what I knew. When you start a dog on a new kibble, we're told to mix the two together while gradually decreasing the old and increasing the new.

So this is what I did when transitioning from kibble to raw — sort of.

1 – Feed Partial Raw, Partial Kibble

While some people will add raw dog food to kibble, I found that the mix of the two made my dogs sick. I read that kibble digests slower than raw, trapping the raw in the digestive system where it begins to decompose and make the dog sick. I don't know how correct this is, but I believed it for a while after Rodrigo vomited all over an area rug after eating a mixed meal. Recently, I learned that kibble creates a different pH in the gut than raw and this is why some dogs get sick when the two foods are mixed in one meal.

We fed our dogs raw dog food in the morning and kibble in the evening until we were out of kibble. This allowed our dogs to get used to eating raw and it allowed us to work out any kinks to feeding raw (ordering, thawing, budget, etc.).

2 – Feed Premade Raw Dog Food

I started our dogs on Darwin's Pet. Darwin's was easy to feed to our dogs and allowed me to take the time to find other sources and learn how to prepare a balanced diet in large batches. With the help of local raw feeders, a few holistic veterinarians, and a ton of reading — our dogs eat 99% prepared raw.

Unfortunately, feeding premade raw is expensive so this isn't a feasible permanent solution for people who are on a budget and/or have multiple big dogs. There was a month when I spent my tax return on premade raw dog food; over $900 in a month!

3 – Go Cold Turkey

When we picked up Scout and Zoey, they were chowing down on Purina – no judgment. On the way home, they ate McDonald's hamburgers (just the meat) — see why I wasn't judging the Purina? And when we made it home 8 or 9 hours later, we fed them their first raw meal and they devoured it.

Our puppies went crazy for their meal. I'd like to think that it's because they knew they were with humans who understood what dogs are supposed to eat. In reality, our puppies were food motivated and hungry after a long day.

Because raw doesn't always come with serving amounts (or ones that make sense), I feed our dogs based on weight. For the 6-week-old Scout and Zoey, we fed them 10% of their current body weight. They were so small, so it was easy to weigh them each week. When their growth slowed down, we fed them 3% of their adult body weight. Today, I judge how much I feed my dogs based on how they look and feel — if I can't feel ribs, for example, then it's time for a diet.

Transitioning a Puppy or Senior to Raw Dog Food

Many people think that a dog has to be a certain age to eat a raw diet. Puppies may be too young and senior dogs may be too old. This is a myth. I started Scout and Zoey on raw at 6 weeks and I know many people who switched their senior dogs to raw and had more time with their beloved pup because of the healthier diet.

The only thing that I would be concerned about are…

- **raw bones** – I don't feel comfortable giving puppies recreational bones while they still have their puppy teeth. I think the bone can be too hard – I have given my puppies bones with a lot of meat and took them away when they meat was gone. I am, however, okay, with giving puppies raw meaty bones like duck necks. With senior dogs that are missing teeth or have extensive dental damage, I would take care with feeding bones, choosing ones that are mostly cartilage and raw meaty bones.

- **liver and heart** — organ meat is very rich and I learned first hand to gradually introduce these foods to a puppy's diet. Feeding too much straight away can lead to diarrhea — explosive diarrhea. I didn't have this issue feeding Darwin's Pet, but I did when I fed my dogs on my own. Part of the problem was also that I was only feeding liver as an offal because at the time I didn't have a source for other secreting organs.

- **how much to feed** — puppies need to eat more than adult dogs and it's suggested that we feed them three to four times a day. I fed Scout and Zoey 10% of their current weight until their growth slowed, then I switched to 3% of their current weight. If you know what your puppy's adult weight will be, you can feed them 3% of that estimate. I didn't make that choice because I worried about not feeding my puppies enough — so 10% worked for us.

5 Things NOT to Do When Transitioning to Raw

1 – DON'T plan to feed your dog only one cut of meat — a balanced raw food diet is 80/10/5/5 — 80% muscle meat, 10% bone, 5% liver, and 5% offal. You can gradually add offal, liver, and alternative proteins to a dog's diet. However, feeding one cut of meat — chicken thighs or ground beef — **for an extended period of time** isn't recommended.

2 – DON'T accept raw recipes from strangers — you'll come across many people who will helpfully give you raw dog food recipes. Do not accept them unless you are prepared to research the ingredients. Are they okay for your dog (some dogs have food allergies)? Can you source the ingredients and, if not, can you find acceptable substitutions? If a recipe is overly complicated, then it's not a good transition recipe.

3 – DON'T feed your dog cooked bones — while feeding bones is an important part of a raw diet for dogs, feeding bones can also be somewhat daunting. If your dog isn't interested in eating recreational bones or raw meaty bones, then you can grind them in their meal and give your dogs bully sticks and a host of other chews that are safe or dogs. Cooked bones can splinter and cause internal damage that can be fatal.

4 – DON'T switch to raw feeding on a whim — if you're still feeding a kibble diet, you can add fresh vegetables, sardines, and mussels, and bone broth to your dog's diet to make it healthier. You can also transition to premade raw dog food which will allow you to improve your dog's diet while giving you the time to research what your dog needs, where to source your ingredients, and anything else you need to know about feeding your dog a raw diet.

5 – DON'T allow others to scare you away — whether it's veterinarians who swear that raw feeding is dangerous or raw feeders who swear that you're doing it wrong; don't allow others to scare you away from feeding your dog a better diet. I had to develop a thick skin when I started down the journey to becoming a raw feeder. There will always be people who will want to tell you that you're wrong — it's your job to decipher the folks who are being helpful (usually they are sharing their experience) and the people who are just being negative (they usually share nothing but judgment).

Understanding Your Dog and Raw Feeding

Letting Your Dog Be Your Guide

My dogs are good at communicating when a meal isn't working for them. In the past, Scout has stepped away from chicken (I had him tested and he has a chicken intolerance) and Rodrigo has stepped away from a meal too high in beef (he's intolerant). When we're learning about raw feeding, we're being clobbered with a lot of information — don't forget to involve your dog in this new diet. You can learn a lot from your best friend too.

UNDERSTANDING YOUR DOG WHEN FEEDING A RAW FOOD DIET

One mistake I see many new raw feeders make is not adjusting the "rules" of raw feeding to their dog. While it's great to learn from more experienced raw feeders, it's important to adjust some of the rules to meet our dogs' needs. In this post, I'm going to share a few ways I've made the "rules" work for my dogs.

START RAW FEEDING WITH CHICKEN

The Rule: I've been told that when we start feeding our dogs a raw food diet, we should start with chicken. I think this is because it's readily available, affordable, and easy for dogs to digest. I know plenty of people who feed a raw diet that is at least 50% chicken to their dogs.

My Rule: Rodrigo and Scout are allergic to chicken. Chicken is a natural inflammatory food and not the best option for dogs with food/environmental allergies or joint pain. Chicken aggravates allergies, makes my dogs itchy, and screws up their tummy. I feed duck instead of chicken. Read the upcoming chapter on Warming Foods, Cooling Foods, and Raw Feeding to learn more about why chicken doesn't work for my dogs.

HOW MUCH I FEED OUR DOGS

The Rule: According to raw food calculators, I should feed our dogs 2.5-3% of their body weight per day; less if I want them to lose weight, more if I want them to gain weight or if they are very active.

My Rule: Rodrigo has a very high metabolism and he's an active dog; he eats about 4% of his body weight. I knew that this was unusual and scheduled a veterinarian appointment for a check up and our vet signed off on how much he was eating. Recently, since adding a pancreas supplement and fermented foods to his diet, I've been able to reduce the amount I feed him slightly.

BARF MODEL RAW DOG FOOD

The Rule: In my research about the BARF model of raw feeding, I see many people instruct us to reduce the amount of muscle meat in a dog's diet, replacing it with vegetables, and dairy. There are other people who suggest that we should also increase the bone in the diet.

My Rule: Reducing the muscle meat and increasing the bone didn't seem right to me, so I feed my dogs 80/10/5/5 (Prey Model) and add organic fruits, vegetables, dairy, and supplements.

CARBS IN RAW DOG FOOD

The Rule: Some people believe that we should remove all carbs from a dog's diet and disagree with the addition of fruits, vegetables, and honey (added for allergies) to a dog's raw diet. Carbs break down into fat when they're not burned off and into sugar which feeds cancer cells. Dogs get all the energy they need from the meat in their diet.

My Rule: While I understand the need to reduce carbs from a dog's raw diet, I don't think all carbs are bad for dogs, therefore, I have chosen not to add grains or high starch foods to my dogs' raw meals.

FATS IN RAW DOG FOOD

The New Rule: Lately, the raw feeding community has been scratching their collective heads as we take in the new rules about balancing fat in a dog's diet. The new information tells us to match fatty acids to the right protein. Below is a chart of which oils I should add based on the proteins I feed to my dogs:

Protein	Ruminant?	Appropriate Fats / Oil
Beef	Y	Hempseed Oil, Walnut Oil, Fish Oil, Sardines
Bison	Y	Hempseed Oil, Walnut Oil, Fish Oil, Sardines
Duck	N	Chia Seeds/Oil, Flax Seed/Oil, Sardines
Elk	Y	Hempseed Oil, Walnut Oil, Fish Oil, Sardines
Emu	N	Unclear
Fish	N	No Oil Necessary
Goat	Y	Hempseed Oil, Walnut Oil, Fish Oil, Sardines
Moose	Y	Hempseed Oil, Walnut Oil, Fish Oil, Sardines
Pheasant	N	Chia Seeds/Oil, Flax Seed/Oil, Sardines
Pork	N	Unclear
Quail	N	Chia Seeds/Oil, Flax Seed/Oil, Sardines
Sheep	Y	Hempseed Oil, Walnut Oil, Fish Oil, Sardines
Venison	Y	Hempseed Oil, Walnut Oil, Fish Oil, Sardines

My Rule: When it comes to the new information on adding fat to my dogs' diet, I'm going to stick with what I'm doing and adjust slowly as I learn more. **Currently, I alternate my dogs' proteins weekly, breaking up each switch with a green tripe day. By doing this, the fats in my dogs diet are balanced without the need for additional oils/seeds.**

Although I trust the sources for this new information on balancing fats, it's important to me that I do homework to see how this change will impact the diet and health of my dogs, find quality sources for the new fats, and seamlessly incorporate them into their diet.

Make Your Own Raw Feeding Rules

While I believe that we should start with the basics of raw feeding — 80/10/5/5 – I don't think we should blindly follow things we read in Facebook groups, on blogs, or in books. When we take the time to understand what our dogs need, we can better adapt to new information, incorporating what we're learning into our dogs' diet.

Despite how far I've come over the past four years, I am always learning and excited when something clicks for my dogs. It can be frustrating when new information flips my diet upside down, making me feel like I have to go back to the beginning, but deep down I know that this is all going to help me raise healthier dogs that live longer lives.

Vaccinations, Vegetables, and Raw Feeding

Vaccinations and Raw Feeding

What do vaccinations have to do with raw feeding? It was only when I started looking into feeding my dogs something different — something that would help Rodrigo's health issues — that I began to learn about over vaccination and unnecessary vaccinations. These topics go hand in hand with early spay and neuter, and chemical flea and tick repellents.

Over vaccination is a hot topic in the dog lover community with some people promoting the belief that brands and pharmaceutical companies are cornering the market by convincing us that we need to expose our dogs to unnecessary chemicals to keep them healthy and safe. Today, I wonder how much of Rodrigo's health issues can be attributed to a kibble diet, annual vaccinations, and monthly Frontline Plus flea and tick treatments.

MY VACCINATION PROTOCOL

Because I'm not a veterinarian, I'm not going to wax philosophical about the evils of vaccinations. Instead, I'll share my thoughts on vaccinating my dogs and my protocol, which has been approved by my vet, who is more conservative than I am on this topic.

While vaccinating our dogs will protect them against illnesses, I'm not comfortable pumping chemicals that I don't understand into their system. My dogs don't go to a kennel, doggy day care, or the dog park. The only dogs they come into contact with are friends who do vaccinate. Rabies isn't a concern in our state; per several local veterinarians. Therefore, I'm comfortable with my choices.

- My dogs are vaccinated as puppies.
- My dogs receive their one-year boosters.

- My dogs are vaccinated when a risk of contracting an illness arises.

At the time of writing this book, I'm keeping an eye on Leptospirosis because we live in an area with an abundance of wildlife. And I'm watching out for canine flu because of the increasing number of cases in other areas of the country.

If pressured, I will do a titer test and if their blood work shows a lack of antibodies, then I will discuss vaccinations with our holistic veterinarian. However, after decades of experience, he told me that my dogs should be covered for life.

IF I HAD TO VACCINATE MY DOGS

If I had to vaccinate my dogs, I would listen to my vet, because I know that he will prescribe an effective detox protocol for my dogs.

Vegetables and Raw Feeding

Asking if it was okay to bring up the topic of vegetables in a raw feeding group got me kicked out, labeled a trouble maker, and harassed for a couple days by the Admin. Most of the drama I see in the raw feeding community has to do with vegetables — should we or shouldn't we?

WHY WE SHOULDN'T FEED VEGETABLES TO DOGS

- Vegetables are just a filler food and have no nutritional benefit for dogs.

- Wolves shake out the stomach content of their prey, ignoring the digesting plant matter. Visit L. David Mech's site to learn more about his 40 year study of wolves in the wild: http://www.davemech.org/

- Vegetables are difficult for dogs to digest, causing the pancreas to work too hard, which can lead to pancreatitis.

- Replacing raw meat with vegetables is not a balanced diet.

I disagree; sort of.

WHY I FEED MY DOGS VEGETABLES

- I feed my dogs vegetables and fruit because I think they provide nutrients, making their raw diet healthier.

- My dogs aren't wolves and I think it would be wrong to feed them like wolves. Unlike wolves, my dogs have been exposed to kibble, vaccinations, spay and neuter surgeries, and they're domesticated.

- I puree my dogs' vegetables to break the cellular wall, making them easier to digest.

- I feed fermented vegetables to provide a natural probiotic.

I do agree that it's wrong for my dogs to eat less meat and more vegetables unless they are on a diet. When I mix up batches of raw dog food, I follow the 80/10/5/5 (muscle meat/bone/offal/liver) and mix in a batch of pureed organic vegetables and fruit.

VEGETABLES AND FRUIT I FEED TO MY DOGS

I created a veggie mix with the help of my veterinarian (see image above); however, I don't always add this to my dogs' raw meals when I'm making a batch. Every other weekend, I puree the following produce, buying organic when I can:

- 2 bundles of kale

- 2 bundles of spinach or collard greens

- 2 bundles of parsley

- 4 zucchini (6 if they're small)

- 1 or 2 celery leaf stalks (not the individual celery)

- 1 or 2 carrots with greens*

- 2 or 3 apples
- 1 package of blueberries

*I have been cutting back on adding carrots, choosing to add hydrated Olewo carrots instead because they support digestive health and skin and coat health, without the glycemic load of fresh carrots.

GMOS AND RAW FEEDING

Although there is a lot of chatter about the health consequences of genetically modified vegetables and fruit. When it comes to my diet, I'm under no illusion that I haven't been happily eating genetically modified foods for years.

While I'm not worried about my own health, I do wonder if there will be an impact on my dogs. At the moment, they have little exposure to genetically modified foods. The reason I want to avoid GMOs in their diet is because (1) they're a different breed and I don't know the long term impact to their health and (2) they live a shorter life and if there is a possibility GMOs can be harmful, I'd like to avoid them when possible.

For me, the jury is still out on the risks of GMOs and my dogs. But I know this will not always be the case.

Warming Foods, Cooling Foods, and Raw Feeding

Warming and Cooling Foods for Dogs

When I was trying to figure out how to give Rodrigo relief from his food and environmental allergies, I came across a site that discussed warming and cooling foods. Chinese medicine teaches us that foods have hot, warming, cooling, and neutral characteristics. I learned that keeping these characteristics in mind can help alleviate inflammation in my dogs.

I didn't understand that feeding Rodrigo a kibble diet was the biggest trigger for his allergies. The ingredients in the kibble act as an inflammatory, worsening joint pain, digestive issues, and allergies.

Rodrigo is a "hot" dog and Sydney is a "cold" dog.

Characteristics of a "Hot" Dog	Characteristics of a "Cold" Dog
they seek out cool places to sleep and rest	they seek out warm places to sleep and rest
they may be hot to the touch	they are relaxed and calm
they pant even when at rest	they love blankets and snuggling
they suffer from allergies	they exhibit a lack of appetite at times
they may have red skin and eyes	
they may show signs of anxiety	

Once I learned about the characteristics of "hot" and "cold" dogs, I realized that the food that I feed them can offer relief or irritate health issues. For example, lamb is a hot food and when Rodrigo eats too much, he stays up half of the night panting and uncomfortable. However, Sydney can eat lamb all week long.

Being "hot" doesn't mean that Rodrigo can't eat the protein; instead, I mix it with a cooling food, like duck meat or only feed the protein in the winter and spring. This may seem complicated, but it's easy and a useful tool when feeding dogs (but not the rule). The following are foods that I feed to my dogs and their characteristics. For a complete list, visit HerbSmithInc.com.

Neutral Foods	Cooling Foods	Warming Foods	Hot Foods
Pork Liver	Duck	Pheasant	Lamb
Pork Kidneys	Rabbit	Mussel	Venison
Quail	Celery	Sweet Potato	Alpaca*
Tripe	Kelp	Goats Milk	Emu*
Bison	Mushroom	Turmeric	Kangaroo*
Sardines	Spirulina		
Mackerel	Apple		
Green Beans			
Shiitake Mushrooms			

*These foods are added to the columns based on Rodrigo's reaction to them.

Warming Foods, Cooling Foods, and Raw Feeding

While it's tempting to remove foods from a dog's diet because we suspect that they identify as “hot” or “cold,” it's important to remember that each dog is different and I feeding a variety of proteins helps alleviate these symptoms as well. I won't remove lamb and venison from Rodrigo's diet, instead, I'll combine them with a cooling protein or limit the amount he eats to keep him comfortable.

MORE FOOD CHARACTERISTICS FOR RAW FEEDERS

Yin Tonifying Foods	Blood Tonic Foods	Foods that Reverse Phlegm	Foods that Reverse Dampness
Signs of a Yin deficiency include panting (especially at night), seeking out cool places, red eyes, and restlessness.	**Signs of a blood deficiency include pale gums, dry/flaky skin, dry/cracked paws, tiring easily, and anemia.**	**Signs of phlegm include a greasy coat, a strong dog smell, hot spots, excessive eye discharge.**	**Signs of dampness include stiffness (especially in cold weather), obesity and loose stool.**
The following foods help…			
Duck	Heart	Kelp	Sardines
Rabbit	Liver	Shiitake Mushrooms	Mackerel
Pork Kidney	Pork	Apples	Celery
Sardines	Sardines		Mushrooms
Spirulina	Kelp		Pumpkin
	Parsley		
	Spinach		

Source: HerbSmithInc.com

Food Energetics and Raw Feeding

Food energetics can seem overwhelming for someone new to raw feeding. We have to think of sourcing, storage, budget, supplements, balancing fats, and now the characteristics of food. Instead of becoming overwhelmed, I slowed down and started with what I knew — lamb meat wasn't a good fit for Rodrigo. As I gained more experience, I began to combine lamb with duck and Rodrigo was fine for a couple of days. He can eat a venison (hot) / duck (cool) blend daily with no issues.

Take your time and incorporate what you can when you're ready. I've used the above lists to help me choose proteins, supplements, and other ingredients for my dogs, which has made raw feeding easier.

eXamining Dog Poop and Raw Feeding

Raw Feeders are Obsessed with Dog Poop

If you belong to a raw feeding group, then you've seen pictures of dog poop. I've had them texted to me, emailed to me, messaged to me. I am SICK of looking at pictures of dog poop. But I get it. One of the benefits of feeding raw is smaller, less smelly dog poop because dogs are utilizing all the nutrients in their food. I saw poop improvement quickly with all of my dogs; Rodrigo's poop became smaller once I started adding a pancreas supplement to his diet and continued to be healthy when I transitioned to fermented foods (vegetables, fish stock, kefir).

At my house, I'm in charge of cleaning up the yard and this works for us because I use this time to see how the dogs are doing. You can learn a lot from dog poop and after years of feeding raw and cleaning the yard, I can tell you which poop belongs to which dog – I'm a rock star.

I clean the dogs' yard daily or every other day. In the winter, I'm outside with a headlamp, flashlight, a lined bucket, and a shovel cleaning the yard. The job never ends.

WHAT I LOOK FOR IN DOG POOP

What I want to see when I'm cleaning the yard is a few piles of small, brown poops. The shade of brown depends on what they're eating — duck creates lighter poop, venison creates darker poop.

My expertise in my dogs' poop was born from Rodrigo's digestive issues. Keeping watch on his poop let me know if he was having a gut flare up or if a protein wasn't working for him. Below is what I used to see with Rodrigo:

Big Poop – Rodrigo's poop was always bigger than the other dogs. I was happy that it was solid more consistently than on kibble and figured that he would never have smaller, raw fed poop because of his gut issues. So I didn't worry too much about it.

White or Light Grey "Soft Serve" Poop – When Rodrigo's poop was white or light gray, it meant that the protein he was eating wasn't working well. He can't eat chicken, turkey, guinea hen, and beef. He can eat green beef tripe with no issues, however, I usually mix the tripe with another protein.

Many people see white poop and think, "too much bone," that isn't the case with Rodrigo. His white poop would be large and soft. If there is too much bone in the diet, in my experience, the poops are white or light in color, hard and sometimes crumble quickly.

My other dogs don't always have perfect poop either and what I occasionally see includes:

Soft Poop with Mucus – This is usually Scout and means that he has an irritated gut. I usually see this if he has too much tripe or if he's swallowed too much pond water when swimming. If it lasts more than 48 hours, I call our veterinarian, especially if combined with a change in behavior (e.g., listlessness, lack of appetite).

Hard Crumbly Poop – Raw fed poops become white and break down quickly, but when fresh poop is crumbling, then there is too much bone in the food.

WHEN DOG POOP RAISES A RED FLAG

My dogs' poop hasn't raised red flags in a long time — knock on wood. However, the following signs will warrant a call to the veterinarian. This is NOT an exhaustive list.

Black, Tarry Dog Poop – this signifies blood higher up in the digestive tract which is scary to me.

Excessive Diarrhea – my dogs have occasional diarrhea or loose stool, but if this goes on for days and there is no sign of easing up, then I'm calling the vet.

Lots of Mucus on the Poop – while mucus on poop is something I see from time to time, if I see a lot of mucus on poop daily, then I worry that there might be something more going on in the digestive tract.

Grey Poop that Doesn't Clear Up – Rodrigo had gray poop once and I panicked and called his nutritionist. She told me to give it a day to see if it clears up; if it doesn't, then it means something is wrong with his bile ducts. It cleared up in less than a day.

HOME REMEDIES FOR DIARRHEA

As I stated, dogs sometimes get diarrhea and it's just a temporary thing and nothing to freak out about. If you are new to feeding raw or raising a dog, I suggest that you err on the side of caution. If you're concerned, call your veterinarian.

Disclaimer: I am not a veterinarian or a nutritionist.

1 – Olewo Carrots – if one of my dogs has diarrhea or loose stool, I'll add Olewo carrots to 1 to 3 of their next meals. Olewo carrots are grown in the fertile rich soils of Germany. Eons ago, carrots soup made from these carrots cured a ton of children of dysentery. The carrots also saved dogs and puppies being raised by a German breeder. And today, they stop diarrhea, improve digestive health, and skin and coat health in our dogs.

2 – Plain Canned Pumpkin – I always have several cans of canned pumpkin as a back up to the Olewo carrots; if I don't have time to hydrate the carrots, I'll mix two tablespoons of plain canned pumpkin into a meal or feed alone. I do this for two days and usually see improvement in 12 – 24 hours.

3 – Slippery Elm – I have never used slippery elm with my dogs, but every time the conversation of diarrhea comes up in raw feeding groups several people recommend slippery elm. It's suggested that we add 1/2 teaspoon per every 10 pounds of body weight.

When it comes to diarrhea, please keep your veterinarian in the loop. If you don't see improvement within 24 hours of using a home remedy, it's time for a call to the vet.

YouTube Channels for Raw Feeders

YouTube is an Excellent Resource for Raw Feeders

If you're a person who learns through observation, YouTube is an excellent resource. Many raw feeders are sharing their experience, their dog's diet, and demonstrating raw feeding (or making a raw meal) on YouTube.

I subscribe to the following four channels:

1 – Dr. Karen Becker

Everyone in the raw community is familiar with Dr. Karen Becker. The reason I recommend her channel is because she covers all aspects of pet health and nutrition. Dr. Becker is a key contributor to the film Pet Fooled, which was written and directed by Kohl Harrington.

2 – Rodney Habib

Rodney Habib is a well-known pet nutrition vlogger, videographer, and writer. Rodney's passion for feeding our dogs better is inspiring and it's always wonderful to follow someone who does so much research, sharing everything he learns for free. Rodney is currently working on a film about the role of diet in treating and curing canine cancer.

3 – Scott Jay Marshall II aka Dog Dad

Scott Jay Marshall II aka Dog Dad has a great channel where he explores all aspects of raw feeding in a down to earth manner. Scott has a rapidly growing and friendly raw feeding group on Facebook: Raw Feeding 101.

4 – Pet Fooled

Pet Fooled is a film that uncovers shocking truths about the pet food industry. Kohl Harrington wrote and directed Pet Fooled over a six year period, creating an informative film that is educating the pet lover community. I follow Pet Fooled because Kohl has continued the dialogue sparked by his film with a 'Talk to Us' campaign where he speaks openly with pet food brands.

The Zen of a Full Freezer and Raw Feeding

When Raw Gets Complicated, a Full Freezer Gives Me Joy

When it comes to raw feeding, it seems like many people go through the same process.

1. We come to the realization that kibble isn't right for our dogs and we start researching raw.

2. We become overwhelmed by the amount of information, opinions, and suggestions — but we power through.

3. We find a person or a group of people to follow which helps to make learning about raw feeding easier.

4. We become brave enough to start feeding our dogs a raw food diet.

5. A year or so later, we can't remember why we were so afraid to get started.

I'm at #5 — it's hard to remember why I was so afraid to get started and then someone flips out in a raw feeding group because they're right and everyone else is wrong and I suddenly remember why I was afraid.

It was hard in the beginning because it was lonely. I didn't have friends who were feeding raw. Every raw feeding group I joined ended with me leaving (or being kicked out) because the group was more focused on drama and attacks than educating and sharing. I wanted to feed my dogs better, but I didn't know how.

Then someone was kind enough to take time out of their schedule to help me. And four years passed and I make raw dog food while watching the Real Housewives.

WHAT I WISH I KNEW THEN

Four years ago, I wish I knew to let it go and focus on my dogs. I allowed myself to get spun up by strangers, distracting me from the goal of feeding my dogs better. While it took me a while to start building a thick skin and look past the negativity of online strangers, I'm getting there.

Instead of worrying about the opinion of strangers on social media, I focus on the status of my freezer. I love that feeling of a full freezer — organized and packed beautifully after an afternoon of meal prep. I swell up with pride and satisfaction knowing that I accomplished something that I thought was impossible a few years ago.

So if you're struggling with trying to figure out raw and you're feeling intimidated by the groups and the amount of information out there — please know that everyone was there, even the people who act as if they were born with the knowledge. You will reach a point where this begins to make sense.

GETTING PAST THE LEARNING CURVE

Raw feeding began to make sense to me when I stopped listening to everyone and started paying attention to my dogs. By considering their needs, raw feeding became less complicated.

WHAT PROTEINS CAN MY DOGS EAT?

We have four dogs, however, Rodrigo is the dog I think of when making raw meals because he's the dog with the most food sensitivities. If he can't eat it, then I have to ask myself if it's worth giving up freezer space for a protein that my dog can't eat.

Sticking with the proteins that all four of my dogs can eat saves me a lot of time and freezer space. The only time I buy proteins that Rodrigo can't eat is when I can get them for a great deal. I feed Rodrigo something he can eat, and the other dogs get the other protein.

- Duck
- Pork
- Venison
- Emu
- Quail
- Lamb
- Green Beef Tripe

WHAT SUPPLEMENTS DO MY DOGS NEED?

In the beginning, I had a cupboard filled with supplements. I could barely keep them straight and it took me 30 minutes to mix up breakfast or dinner for the dogs. Today, I only have a handful of supplements and give the dogs only what each one needs. I've learned that a lot of the supplements I added either canceled others out, acted as a duplicate, or could be replaced with fresh food.

- Milk Thistle
- Spirulina
- Green Lipped Mussel Powder
- Golden Paste
- Fish Oil
- Kelp
- Canine System Saver

SAVE TIME, SAVE MONEY, FEED RAW

By focusing on my dogs, I have been able to take in what people share in the raw feeding groups, absorbing what will work for my dogs while I disregard the rest. It makes raw feeding less complicated. There will always be days when we get frustrated with the constant flood of information provided — just vent it out with friends (we all understand) and move on. We are doing the best we can with the information we have and the sources within our reach.

When I become frustrated by someone telling me that I'm feeding raw wrong (aka, I'm not doing what they're doing) and when respected leaders tell us that we have to feed raw in life stages while balancing dietary fats, I remind myself that we're always learning and then I walk out to the freezer in the garage and marvel at how organized it is, and then I smile.

Raw Dog Food Recipes

Recipes for Making Raw Dog Food

The following are recipes that I commonly make for my dogs. They include both ground and whole raw recipes, along with a recipe for bone broth, turmeric paste, and a vegetable mix.

Keep in mind that these recipes are for four dogs that weigh between 60-75 pounds. I am sharing them to give you and idea of what you can feed to your dog and you are welcome to adapt them to meet your dog's needs.

Rabbit and Green Tripe/Organ Blend

The rabbit is sourced from a local farm (through our raw food co-op) and the cost is at the higher range for proteins. None of my dogs have an intolerance to rabbit, making it a hit in our home. I wish I could get a different grind; it's finely ground, making it very thick and sticky, a texture that I don't care for in raw food.

My dogs love it and adding a vegetable mix makes it less sticky and easier to manage.

I can buy whole rabbit and grind it myself (it's less expensive), but I'm too much of a coward to deal with whole.

INGREDIENTS:

- 12 pounds of ground whole rabbit
- 2 pounds of green tripe/organ blend (beef heart, lungs, liver, spleen and pancreas with green tripe)
- 2 pounds of vegetable mix (optional)

EQUIPMENT:

- Stainless steel bowls
- Mixing spoons
- Wire masher
- Rubbermaid containers

DIRECTIONS:

I mix all of the ingredients in several huge stainless steel bowls. Once mixed, I transfer the ingredients into Rubbermaid containers and into the fridge and freezer.

The rabbit and green tripe blend are preground. I can feed rabbit and veggies only, however, I decided to add the green tripe/organ blend to give the dogs something new to eat. I use a masher because of the rabbit is very hard to mix otherwise; adding water, vegetables and the green tripe blend makes it a little easier to mix.

The above ingredients do not represent a balanced meal; I took the meal out of balance when I added the green tripe blend, which is optional.

Ground Sardines

I can order whole sardines through our co-op. Rodrigo loves them and will eat them in the yard. They are flash frozen after being caught off the Oregon coast and arrive in 50-pound boxes. I have to partially thaw the box and redistribute into manageable packages.

However, it's a pain in the butt and too much fish to deal with so I purchased a case of sardine chubs (the food comes in a tube form) from Primal Pet Food. This is just sardine grind and looks like a brown mush. It's tempting to wonder if this is really fish, but once you get a whiff, you're sure. Plus, I've ground up fish before and that's close to what it looks like — a brown mush.

It's not very appetizing to me; the dogs love it.

When feeding, I split the dogs' meals in half, giving them 1/2 of the duck/veggie grind (or other grind on hand) and 1/2 of the Primal Pet sardine grind. I mixed it together, added thawed green beans to the girls' meals (they're on a diet), and served with their supplements.

It was a hit!

Green Tripe

My dogs eat green tripe from GreenTripe.com and bison tripe from Darwin's Pet.

Xkaliber is a blend of green tripe, beef muscle meat, beef heart, beef tongue, beef trachea/gullet, and ground bone (not bone meal). GreenTripe.com tells us that this blend is great for younger dogs and serious working dogs. It helps build muscle, bone and stamina. It is also excellent for older dogs if fed a couple of times a week.

The dogs love the Xkaliber.

The food comes in a chub, pre-ground and ready to serve.

INGREDIENTS:

- 6 pounds (3 chubs) of Xkaliber
- 2 pounds of vegetable mix (optional)
- frozen green beans (for the girls, their on a diet)

EQUIPMENT:

No equipment needed; everything can be added to each dog's dish directly from the chub. The vegetable mixes are premade and the frozen green beans are thawed before served.

DIRECTIONS:

I add Xkaliber until each dog's dish is at the appropriate weight. I then add in vegetables and green beans. This week, my dogs are eating pureed vegetables mixed into their raw because I didn't have time to make their Veggie Mix.

This is a balanced raw diet for one week with four big dogs that range from 60 pounds to 75 pounds.

Ground Rabbit

The rabbit I buy for our dogs is sourced from a local farm (through our raw food co-op). It is whole ground rabbit and doesn't require additional organ meat or bone unless I decide to mix in other ingredients.

INGREDIENTS:

- 12 pounds of ground whole rabbit
- 2 pounds of vegetable mix (optional)

EQUIPMENT:

- Stainless steel bowls
- Mixing spoons
- Blender
- Mixer (optional)
- Rubbermaid containers

DIRECTIONS:

I add ground rabbit until each dog's dish is at the appropriate weight. I then add in vegetables and green beans.

The above ingredients will create a balanced meal for three or four days for my four big dogs.

Duck Gizzards

In the grocery store, gizzards are cheap. I remember my mom buying them as a snack. She'd season them and fry them in a pan, which I still do today.

Gizzards for my dogs are more expensive. A lot more expensive. Of course, the ones I buy for myself are chicken. My dogs eat duck. Nothing but the best.

INGREDIENTS:

- 40 pounds of duck wings
- 30 pounds of duck gizzards
- 5 pounds of turkey hearts
- 4 pounds of organ/offal blend by GreenTripe.com (2-2 lb chubs)
- 2 pork liver*
- 8 pork kidneys*
- 5 pounds of vegetables (optional)

* I went heavier on offal and liver this week because I didn't feed enough last week.

EQUIPMENT:

- Stainless steel bowls
- Mixing spoons
- Meat grinder
- Blender
- Mixer (optional)
- Rubbermaid containers

DIRECTIONS:

I grind all of the meat and mix them in several huge stainless steel bowls.

Once mixed, I transfer the ingredients into Rubbermaid containers and into the fridge and freezer.

The above ingredients will create a balanced meal for at least a week for my four big dogs.

Columbia River Guinea Hen

I ordered guinea hen from Columbia River Natural as an alternative to chicken, which I don't feed, because two of my dogs are allergic. Turns out that guinea hen is not a good alternative. The girls did great on the protein, the boys didn't do so hot after a couple days of eating it because it's similar to chicken.

INGREDIENTS:

- 10 pounds of guinea hen by Columbia River Natural
- 2 pounds of organ/offal blend by GreenTripe.com (1-2 lb chubs)
- 2 pounds of a vegetable mix (optional)

EQUIPMENT:

- Stainless steel bowls
- Mixing spoons
- Mixer (optional)
- Rubbermaid containers

DIRECTIONS:

I typically grind all of the meat and mix them in several huge stainless steel bowls. Once mixed, I transfer the ingredients into Rubbermaid containers and into the fridge and freezer. Columbia River Natural pet food comes ground, so this saved me a step.

The vegetable mix can be added while mixing all of the meat or to each meal as you feed your dogs. I do both depending on what I have on hand (and what I remember to do).

The above ingredients will create a balanced meal for at least a week for my four big dogs.

Duck and Turkey

Sometimes I like to blend proteins for my dogs. Rodrigo has trouble eating too much turkey, but he does well with a diet of minimal turkey (like this one) and mostly duck or other poultries like pheasant and quail.

INGREDIENTS:

- 20 pounds of duck wings
- 30 pounds of duck gizzards (or venison when I don't have gizzards)
- 5 pounds of duck hearts (or turkey hearts)
- 10 pounds of turkey scapula meat
- 8 pounds of organ/offal blend by GreenTripe.com (four ground2 lb chubs)
- 5 pounds of a vegetable mix (optional)

EQUIPMENT:

- Stainless steel bowls
- Mixing spoons
- Meat grinder
- Mixer (optional)
- Rubbermaid containers

DIRECTIONS:

I grind all of the meat and mix them in several huge stainless steel bowls. Once mixed, I transfer the ingredients into Rubbermaid containers and into the fridge and freezer.

The vegetable mix can be added while mixing all of the meat or to each meal as you feed your dogs. I do both depending on what I have on hand (and what I remember to do). This week, my dogs are eating very little vegetables in their meal simply because I forgot to thaw out veggie mix. A break here and there doesn't hurt.

The above ingredients will create a balanced meal for at least a week for my four big dogs.

Duck, Emu, and Green Tripe/Organ Blend

The emu is sourced from through our raw food co-op and the cost is at the higher range for proteins. Emu is a "hot" protein, so I only feed it to Rodrigo for two days in a row or I feed it to him with duck wings.

INGREDIENTS:

- 50 pounds of ground emu
- 20 pounds of duck wings
- 8 pounds of green tripe/organ blend (beef heart, lungs, liver, spleen and pancreas with green tripe)
- 3-5 pounds of vegetable mix (optional)

EQUIPMENT:

- Stainless steel bowls
- Mixing spoons
- Wire masher
- Rubbermaid containers

DIRECTIONS:

I mix all of the ingredients in several huge stainless steel bowls. Once mixed, I transfer the ingredients into Rubbermaid containers and into the fridge and freezer.

The emu and green tripe blend are preground.

VEGETABLE MIX:

The vegetable mix can be added while mixing all of the meat or to each meal as you feed your dogs. I do both depending on what I have on hand (and what I remember to do).

The above ingredients represent a balanced meal.

Duck Carcass and Green Tripe/Organ Blend

This year, I discovered the wonders of duck carcass. Scout was showing little interest in his meals so I decided to take a break from ground raw. I ordered a case of duck carcasses from our local raw food co-op. They are the duck torso (no head, legs) with meat, bone, and cartilage. The below is a recipe for two meals (one day) for my dogs.

INGREDIENTS:

- 4 to 6 duck carcasses
- 1/2 pound of green tripe/organ blend (beef heart, lungs, liver, spleen and pancreas with green tripe)
- 2 or 3 ice cubes of vegetable mix, slightly melted (optional)

EQUIPMENT:

- Meat cleaver (optional)
- Cutting board (optional)

DIRECTIONS:

My dogs are fed twice a day. In the morning, they shared 1/2 pound the green tripe/organ blend along with the vegetable ice cubes (slightly melted).

At the time of this meal, we were enjoying a great summer and I fed the dogs their duck carcasses outside in the evening. A duck carcass weighs approximately 11-12 ounces; I use a meat cleaver to cut two carcasses in half to split between the boys because they eat more than my girls.

The above ingredients do not represent a balanced meal, however, this is fine to feed, simply balance your dog's diet over time.

I Forgot to Thaw Raw Meals for My Dogs!!!

It happens; all the time. I bolt awake at 4 am and realize that I forgot to thaw meals for my dogs. If it's a weekend or I have the day off, no problem - I put a few chubs in a bowl of room temperature water and food will be ready in a couple hours.

There are times when I'm not that lucky and this is what I do.

INGREDIENTS:

- Duck necks, slightly thawed
- Freeze-dried raw (I prefer Steve's Real Food, NRG Dehydrated Food, and Vital Essentials Raw)
- Sardines, canned in water with no salt added
- Raw eggs

EQUIPMENT:

- Stainless steel bowls

DIRECTIONS:

I pull a package of duck necks from the freezer and separate four using warm water to melt the ice; I set those four necks in a bowl of room temperature water to being thawing, placing the remainder in the fridge.

I pour the appropriate amount of freeze-dried raw or dehydrated food into the dogs' dishes and add water to hydrate.

At this time, I take my shower, get dressed, do hair and make up, then head back downstairs - 25 minutes.

I add 3 sardines to each dog's hydrated meal along with 1 egg each and 1 duck neck.

The above ingredients do not represent a balanced meal; but it's a healthy raw meal fed in a pinch. Plus, I balance over time.

Bone Broth

Bone broth is fantastic for the immune system, digestive system, and joints. I make a batch at least once a month to add to my dogs' food or feed as a frozen treat in the summer.

BENEFITS OF BONE BROTH FOR DOGS:

- Bone broth promotes a healthy digestive system
- It's great for Rodrigo and Sydney's joints
- It acts as a liver detox, so if you have your dogs on an kibble (no judgment, we all do the best we can), this is an affordable way to give your dog something better. Plus in this chemically laden world, our dogs can use a detox here and there.
- And bone broth is great for sick dogs, because it provides them nutrition when they don't have much of an appetite.

INGREDIENTS (these vary based on what's available):

I source most of my bones through our local raw food co-op; I prefer joint bones with cartilage.

- Bones (turkey, emu, lamb)
- Apple cider vinegar
- 2 cloves of fresh garlic (perfectly safe for dogs)
- Kale, dandelion, or turmeric powder (optional)

EQUIPMENT:

- Slow cooker (takes 24 hours) or pressure cooker (takes 3-4 hours)
- Spoon with ladle (to fish out bones)

- Rubbermaid containers

DIRECTIONS:

I fill my pressure cooker (or slow cooker) with bones, add enough water to cover the bones. I add 1/4 cup of apple cider vinegar and garlic. Cook until finished (slow cooker takes 24 hours, my pressure cooker takes 3-4 hours).

I allow the bone broth to cool for a couple hours or overnight.

I fish out the bones (keep meat in broth) from the broth and spoon broth into Rubbermaid containers to store in the freezer for later use.

I do not buy broth from the grocery store because I don't know what bones were used (I prefer joint bones) and many brands add onions and a lot of salt, which aren't healthy for dogs.

Turmeric Paste aka Golden Paste

I began making golden paste for my dog to help her recover from a partial cruciate tear. Combining golden paste with her joint supplement and food-grade diatomaceous earth resulted in better mobility (running and playing) within 48 hours.

Today, I've replaced the food-grade diatomaceous earth with Canine System Saver and she's back to being a happy, playful girl.

I make my golden paste in large batches, storing the excess in the freezer. It is good in the fridge for 2 weeks.

BENEFITS OF GOLDEN PASTE FOR DOGS:

This is a short list of the benefits of golden paste for dogs:

- Natural detox
- Anti-inflammatory
- Natural antibacterial
- Promotes heart and liver health
- Reduces blood clots that can lead to strokes and heart attacks by thinning the blood
- Promotes digestive health
- Acts as an antioxidant AND it's believed to be able to prevent cancer
- Offers allergy relief
- Helps to prevent cataracts
- Has been used in the treatment of epilepsy

- Natural pain relief
- Natural treatment for diarrhea

INGREDIENTS:

- 3 cups of turmeric powder (I order through our co-op)
- 6 cups of water
- 2 cups of organic coconut oil (or 1 cup of coconut oil and 1 cup of bone broth)
- 3 tablespoons of freshly ground pepper (from a pepper mill)
- 2 tablespoons of Cylon cinnamon

EQUIPMENT:

- Sauce pan
- Stove
- Spoon
- Whisk
- Rubbermaid containers

DIRECTIONS:

Step 1: I slowly warm the water on the lowest heat while I ground the pepper I need.

Step 2: I mix the turmeric powder in with the water and stir until it begins to get thick.

Step 3: I mix in the coconut oil and bone broth, and, finally, the pepper. I turn off the heat and continue to stir.

Step 4: I allow the turmeric paste to cool and transfer into Rubbermaid containers to freeze.

TURMERIC PASTE DOSAGE FOR DOGS

I've read different dosages on several sites. Many people advise to start with small amounts and build up because it can cause loose stool if you feed too much to your dog. Turmeric paste leaves a dog's system quickly, so it should be fed with each meal (more than once a day). I started my dogs off with 1/4 teaspoon in each meal and worked up from there to gauge their tolerance. Ultimately, you want to do 1/4 teaspoon for every 10 pounds of body weight.

- Start by adding 1/4 – 1/2 teaspoon of golden paste to each meal
- Every 5-7 days, increase the dosage a small amount
- Once you notice pain relief, increased mobility, or a decrease in tumor size (yeah, I read this could happen and I'm blown away) — you've found your maintenance dosage

For our dogs that don't have any pre-existing health issues (joints and digestive), I stick with the lower dosage of 1/4 – 1/2 teaspoon per meal, because more gives them diarrhea.

Veggie Mix

My dogs' veterinarian recommended that I begin adding more vegetables to my dogs' diet to help Sydney lose weight. He gave me a list of vegetables and fruit that were a good fit for my dogs and, with the help of other raw feeders, I created a vegetable mix.

BENEFITS OF VEGETABLES FOR DOGS:

While some raw feeders don't feel that vegetables are a natural part of a dog's diet, I disagree.

- Vegetables provide antioxidants that are known to fight off cancer.
- Vegetables help balance a dog's system, keeping it from being too acidic or too alkaline.
- Vegetables provide additional nutrients when fed pureed or fermented.
- Fermented vegetables offer a natural source of probiotics; Note: this isn't a recipe for fermented vegetables.
- Vegetables provide fiber to help with digestion.
- Vegetables can help an overweight dog feel full when on a diet.

INGREDIENTS (these vary based on what's available):

I source most of my organic vegetables and fruits from the grocery store. I alternate the vegetables I add, only using two greens (i.e., kale and spinach, or spinach and collard greens).

- 2 bundles of kale
- 2 bundles of spinach or collard greens
- 2 bundles of parsley

- 4 zucchini (6 if they're small)
- 1 or 2 celery leaf stalks (not the individual celery)
- 1 or 2 carrots with greens or hydrated Olewo carrots
- 2 or 3 apples
- 1 package of blueberries
- 5 cloves of fresh garlic (yes, this is safe for my dogs in this amount)
- 1 or 2 packages of freeze dried mushrooms — shiitake, crimini, portobello (optional)
- 1 inch of ginger (optional)
- Apple cider vinegar (optional)
- Bone broth (optional)
- Turmeric paste (optional)

EQUIPMENT:

- Blender or food processor
- Knife
- Cutting board
- Large stainless steel bowls
- Large spoon or ladle for mixing
- Rubbermaid containers or ice cube trays

DIRECTIONS:

I chop up the vegetables and fruit to make it easier to puree in the blender. I fill each large bowl with the blended vegetables and fruit, leaving room to add in bone broth and turmeric paste.

I pour the mixture into Rubbermaid containers or ice cube trays to freeze. Or, if I'm prepping future raw meals, I'll mix the vegetable mix in with the raw blend.

If you don't have time to make bone broth, there is premade bone broth available at some local pet stores. I do not buy broth from the grocery store because I don't know what bones were used (I prefer joint bones) and many brands add onions and salt, which aren't healthy for dogs.

Please note: this is not a recipe to create fermented vegetables.

Quick Reference Guide

WHAT TO FEED A DOG

Muscle Meat	Raw Bones	Liver	Offal
80%	10%	5%	5%
e.g. Venison, Lamb, Goat, Rabbit, Pheasant, Quail, Duck, Elk, Emu	e.g. Duck Necks, Lamb Necks	Liver	e.g. Pancreas, Spleen, Kidneys

The above chart represents foods that I feed to my dogs; there are many more options available.

HOW MUCH TO FEED A DOG

Dogs are fed 2-4% of their body weight per day, split between two meals. It's recommended that we start with 2% if our dog is fat, feed 2.5-3% to maintain a dog's current weight, and feed more to help a dog gain weight. Puppies are feed 10% of their current body weight or 3% of their estimated adult body weight per day, split between three meals.

It's important to note that the percentages above are a starting point. Every dog is different.

If you find that your dog is gaining too much weight or losing too much weight, adjust their meal accordingly.

ORGANS VS. OFFAL

To feed a "balance" raw food diet, we're advised to feed 80% muscle meat, 10% bone, 5% liver, and 5% offal, which are secreting organs. As humans, we consider chicken hearts and gizzards organ mean, however, in raw feeding, they are considered "meat," not organs.

The below chart will help you differentiate between meat and offal when planning your dog's raw meals.

Organs Fed as Muscle Meat	Organs Fed as Offal	Other Cuts of Meat Fed as Muscle
Heart	**Pancreas**	**Green Tripe**
Gizzard	**Kidney**	**Trachea**
Lung	**Spleen**	**Tongue**
	Testicles	
	Brain	

RAW BONES THAT WORK WITH MY DOGS

Raw Meaty Bones	Recreational Bones
Duck Necks	**Beef Knuckle Bones**
Lamb Necks	**Beef Knee Caps**
Turkey Necks	**Buffalo Knuckle Bones**
Duck Frames	

I know raw feeders who give their dogs rib bones. Rodrigo is a strong, chewer and when he tried rib bones, they splintered too much and he attempted to swallow a long shard which took that bone off the list in our home.

WARMING AND COOLING FOODS

Neutral Foods	Cooling Foods	Warming Foods	Hot Foods

Pork Liver	Duck	Pheasant	Lamb
Pork Kidneys	Rabbit	Mussel	Venison
Quail	Celery	Sweet Potato	Alpaca*
Tripe	Kelp	Goats Milk	Emu*
Bison	Mushroom	Turmeric	Kangaroo*
Sardines	Spirulina		
Mackerel	Apple		
Green Beans			
Shiitake Mushrooms			

*These foods are added to the columns based on Rodrigo's reaction to them.

CPSIA information can be obtained
at www.ICGtesting.com
Printed in the USA
LVHW090149260721
693672LV00008B/38